Protected

Protected

Birth Control's Remarkable Story and Uncertain Future

Katherine Quimby

BLOOMSBURY ACADEMIC
NEW YORK • LONDON • OXFORD • NEW DELHI • SYDNEY

BLOOMSBURY ACADEMIC
Bloomsbury Publishing Inc, 1359 Broadway, New York, NY 10018, USA
Bloomsbury Publishing Plc, 50 Bedford Square, London, WC1B 3DP, UK
Bloomsbury Publishing Ireland, 29 Earlsfort Terrace, Dublin 2, D02 AY28, Ireland

BLOOMSBURY, BLOOMSBURY ACADEMIC and the Diana logo are trademarks of Bloomsbury Publishing Plc

First published in the United States of America 2025

Copyright © Katherine Quimby, 2025

Cover image © Front cover image of birds © iStock.com/tigerstrawberry, image of pomegranate © iStock.com/deepfuze

All rights reserved. No part of this publication may be: i) reproduced or transmitted in any form, electronic or mechanical, including photocopying, recording or by means of any information storage or retrieval system without prior permission in writing from the publishers; or ii) used or reproduced in any way for the training, development or operation of artificial intelligence (AI) technologies, including generative AI technologies. The rights holders expressly reserve this publication from the text and data mining exception as per Article 4(3) of the Digital Single Market Directive (EU) 2019/790.

Bloomsbury Publishing Inc does not have any control over, or responsibility for, any third-party websites referred to or in this book. All internet addresses given in this book were correct at the time of going to press. The author and publisher regret any inconvenience caused if addresses have changed or sites have ceased to exist, but can accept no responsibility for any such changes.

A catalog record for this book is available from the Library of Congress

ISBN: HB: 979-8-8818-0469-5
ePDF: 979-8-7651-6516-4
eBook: 979-8-8818-0470-1

Typeset by Deanta Global Publishing Services, Chennai, India
Printed and bound in the United States of America

For product safety related questions contact productsafety@bloomsbury.com.

To find out more about our authors and books visit www.bloomsbury.com and sign up for our newsletters.

For champions of reproductive health

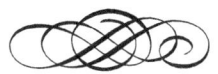

Contents

Disclaimer ix

Introduction: Why Birth Control? Why Now? 1
1 In the Beginning: When Crocodile Poop Was Your Best Option for Birth Control 15
2 Strange Bedfellows: The Complicated History of Birth Control, Religion, and Politics 33
3 From Obscene to Ostracized: Population Control and the Origins of "Family Planning" 51
4 It Takes Two: Why We Don't Have a Birth Control Pill for Men—and How Close We Are to Getting It 59
5 The Magic Pill: How Two Women Changed the World Forever 73
6 Shocking and Shameful: How Birth Control Has Been Used for Evil 89
7 More Methods, More Problems: The Misuse of Long-Term, Highly Effective Birth Control 101
8 The Obstacle Course: It Can Be Really, Really Hard to Get Birth Control 115
9 Today's Specials Are: The Menu of Birth Control Options and the Many Factors That Might Influence Which One Will Work Best for You 125

10 Not Just for Pregnancy Prevention: How Birth Control Helps with Period Pain, Acne, Cancer, and More 147
11 Changing Lives, Changing Societies: How Birth Control Has Changed the World 165
12 On the Cutting Edge: What the Future Holds for Birth Control 177
13 Birth Control Needs You 187

Keep the Discussion Going 191
Acknowledgments 193
Notes 195
References 199
Index 241

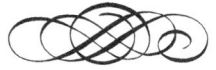

Disclaimer

This book does not provide medical advice. The content is for informational purposes only. This book is not intended to be a substitute for professional medical advice, diagnosis, or treatment. Always seek the advice of your physician or other qualified healthcare provider.

Introduction

Why Birth Control? Why Now?

Birth control matters. For everyone. For as long as people have been having sex, they have wanted to prevent the sometimes inopportune result: pregnancy. In fact, few experiences are *as* universal as using birth control. It's an experience that ties us together across geography, demographics, and generations going back thousands of years. Today, over 99 percent of sexually experienced American women between the ages of fifteen and forty-four have used at least one method of birth control ever in their lives.[1] And while I'm going to mostly focus on the United States, birth control matters across the globe, where an estimated 966 million women are currently using some method of birth control. And that's just women, who aren't even the only ones who use birth control. People of all genders use birth control for a whole range of reasons.

Most of us will use more than one method of birth control in our lifetimes. The journey to find a birth control method that works can be a long, drama-filled story fit for a Netflix special (am I the only one who thinks this would be interesting TV?) Maybe your birth control saga was similar to mine. I was first prescribed the birth control patch because even as a teenager I couldn't figure out how to swallow pills (yes, I know that's weird). After I did finally figure out a pill-swallowing technique, I switched to the pill, trying a few kinds to sort out side effects. I got tired of the pill in college and wanted something I didn't have to deal with every day, so I switched again to the ring. I spent $50 a month for the ring, which I paid for by working a $7.75 minimum wage job at my college dining hall.

When I was in college, the Affordable Care Act was passed, and with it came insurance coverage for birth control. Birth control became more affordable for a lot of Americans, myself included. I could finally rationalize getting the birth control implant, which would previously have cost several hundreds of dollars out of my pocket but would now be entirely covered by my insurance. The birth control implant doesn't work for everyone, but it has worked for me. I've used two all the way to the end of their shelf life of three years (although more recent research shows they are effective for up to five). I've also had them removed in order to get pregnant two times, and the midwives who assisted me during my deliveries were kind enough to place a new implant in my upper arm before I even left the hospital.

By my tally, I'm now on my fifth type of birth control. And that doesn't even take into account the fact that there were a few brands of pills tried over the years (there are so many different kinds!), as well as condoms and the occasional morning-after pill which have also made appearances on this Netflix special. With all that factored in, I think I might even have hit double digits. Is that a hint of pride in my voice? Yes, yes, it is. I'm passionate about this stuff!

Maybe you were fortunate to find something quickly that has worked for you for ages. Maybe you've used different types of methods here and there, but you're not using anything right now. Maybe you're still looking for something that works for you. Many people spend *decades* using some sort of birth control to help build the family size they want—whether the number of children is zero or anything more than that. Excluding the time I spent pregnant, I've been on birth control for my *entire adult life*—and there's a good chance you have been, too.

At any given time, about nine in ten American women who are sexually active and not actively trying to get pregnant are using a birth control method. This has been fairly constant for decades. There are many reasons why one in ten are *not* using birth control, such as concerns about side effects, ambivalence about pregnancy (maybe they're not actively seeking pregnancy but wouldn't mind if they became pregnant), only having same-sex partners, or simply not wanting to be on birth control. While preventing pregnancy is the main reason people use birth control, one in five people using birth control say they use it for a different reason, like managing periods or medical conditions. Preventing sexually transmitted infections (STIs) is another big reason why someone might use birth control, and specifically only condoms can help do that. Probably for that reason, condoms are among the most commonly used types of birth control, along with pills and sterilization (See Table 0.1).

Most discussion about birth control centers around women. But people of all genders use birth control. Preventing pregnancy is something that a lot of people care about—not just women. Some transgender men to use birth control to prevent pregnancy and manage symptoms of gender dysphoria. And in 2017, the Male Contraceptive Initiative fielded an online survey of 1,500 males ages eighteen to forty-four living in the United States. More than 80 percent of them reported currently trying to prevent pregnancy, and—this is where it gets interesting—80 percent *also* felt sole or shared responsibility for pregnancy prevention. There is a big opportunity for men to participate more fully in pregnancy prevention.

There is some variation in who uses birth control, for sure. Different people have different preferences when it comes to birth control, and

Table 0.1 Percentage of Women Who Have Used Each Type of Birth Control

Birth Control Method	% of Women Ever Used	% of Women Used in Last 12 Months
Pill	71	33
Condoms	65	32
Sterilization—Tubal ligation ("Tubes tied") or hysterectomy	23	*
Emergency contraception (like Plan B pills)	22	7
IUD	21	19
Fertility awareness-based method	19	15
Injection	16	4
Sterilization—Vasectomy	15	*
Implant	8	5
Patch	8	2
Ring	8	3
Other	8	4

Source: Frederiksen, Brittni, Usha Ranji, Michelle Long, Karen Diep, and Alina Salganicoff. "Contraception in the United States: A Closer Look at Experiences, Preferences, and Coverage | KFF." KFF, November 18, 2022.
Notes: *Since sterilization procedures are permanent, they were not asked about separately in the past twelve months; Respondents could report multiple methods used.

some people can get birth control more easily than other people. But across the board, about 80–90 percent of women use birth control across race, marital status, income level, age, sexual orientation, and insurance status. Ben Franklin famously said that nothing in the world is certain except death and taxes. Well, in any given year, 72 percent of Americans pay federal income taxes, so in fact, he would have been more accurate if he had said the only certainties in life are death *and birth control.*

Preventing pregnancy is, understandably, a priority for most of us. As someone with two kids, I am *very, very* interested in not being pregnant. It turns out I am not alone in this. Among all women ages between eighteen and forty-nine who are not currently trying to get pregnant, 70 percent of us say that avoiding pregnancy is important, and that increases to 81 percent among women currently using birth control.

For how pervasive and fundamental birth control is, it's curious how little attention it gets from us in our daily lives. Birth control isn't something we tend to talk about outside of the privacy of our own homes or doctors' offices. And sometimes it's difficult to talk about birth control even in *those* settings. Maybe that's because we think it's controversial and want to avoid landing in the middle of a contentious debate. Maybe it's because we feel we don't know enough about birth control to talk about it accurately and effectively. More likely, it's because to talk about birth control is to talk about the taboo topics of sex and medical conditions for which birth control is used to treat. These topics can be uncomfortable. But I say, it's time to be uncomfortable.

Now is the time for birth control to get out of the shadows of our own lives. We simply can't afford for birth control to be a taboo topic any longer. While this is an exciting time for birth control—with a larger, more comprehensive menu of methods than ever before—it's also a concerning time for birth control. The right to abortion is gone. It's already hard for a lot of people to get birth control. Laws that restrict birth control will make it even harder for people—maybe even you—to get the health care they need.

There's Never Been a More Important Time to Care about Birth Control

On February 16, 2024, the Alabama Supreme Court issued a decision that shocked the country.

The case involved three couples who had gone through in vitro fertilization (IVF) treatment at a fertility clinic in Mobile, Alabama. The couples were storing their fertilized eggs (or "embryos") at the clinic while they prepared to transfer them in the hopes of becoming pregnant.

But in December 2020, a patient entered the clinic through an unsecured door and opened up the tanks containing the couples' fertilized eggs. (I imagine this like a scene from a Mission Impossible movie—a masked man dodging security lasers—but in reality, it was probably much less dramatic.) Unfortunately for him, he didn't realize that the tank was kept at sub-freezing temperatures. When he reached in to grab the container with the fertilized eggs, the extreme cold burned his hand, causing him to drop the container to the ground. The fertilized eggs were destroyed.

Three couples whose fertilized eggs were destroyed filed a lawsuit against the fertility clinic. They claimed that the clinic should be held responsible for the wrongful deaths of minors based on an Alabama state law dating back to 1872 (almost one hundred years before IVF existed). The Alabama Supreme Court ruled in the couples' favor, saying that the Wrongful Death of a Minor Act applied "to all unborn children without limitation. And that includes unborn children who are not located in utero at the time they are killed." For reference, a fertilized egg is a *tiny* mass of cells, no bigger than a freckle.

Fertility clinics in Alabama immediately halted their IVF services. While the details of the case were unusual—it's not often that patients find their way into what should be a secured storage unit—there is always a possibility that fertilized eggs can be damaged or destroyed during IVF, and fertility clinics didn't want to risk a lawsuit.

Some patients in the middle of treatment were forced to leave Alabama to find care in another state. After enduring three miscarriages within a nine-month period, Gabrielle Goidel had invested more than $20,000 into IVF and was just a few days away from undergoing an egg retrieval when the Alabama Supreme Court decision came down. After desperately calling around to IVF clinics begging them to help her finish her treatment, she packed her bags and got on a plane to Texas, hoping to continue her treatment there.

Elizabeth Goldman was also deep in the middle of her treatment. Born without a uterus, there was a time she thought she would never be able to get pregnant. Through a uterus transplant program at the University of Alabama at Birmingham and with the help of IVF, she was able to carry a daughter in a transplanted uterus. But a transplanted uterus must be removed after a couple of years to avoid long-term damage to the body. A delay, like the one caused by the Alabama Supreme Court, threatened Goldman's plans to carry a second child in the short time frame that she could safely do so.

IVF is a time-sensitive process, not to mention a process that can take an enormous physical and emotional toll. The uncertainty around if, when, and how they would be able to complete their treatment left people confused, devastated, and frustrated.

There was a national outcry in response to the ruling. People who received IVF treatment, along with the children born to parents who used IVF, spoke out about how taking away IVF was cruel, unfair, and inhumane. If people want to create families, they said, what right does the Alabama Supreme Court have to take that away?

Three weeks later, the Alabama legislature passed a law in response to the public backlash. The new law protected IVF patients and providers from legal liability. This was comforting enough that the fertility clinics in Alabama could start up their IVF services again. But the law failed to address the issue at the root of the ruling: that the state's Wrongful Death of a Minor Act extends to fertilized eggs.

While all of this unfolded in Alabama, people across the country looked on with concern. There are over a million and a half frozen fertilized eggs across the country. Nearly 250,000 people undergo IVF each year, and about 2 percent of all babies born in the United States are conceived with IVF. Looking at the Alabama case, people wondered, will my state follow Alabama's lead? Will I be able to have the baby that I want to have?

Now, you might be wondering, what the heck does IVF have to do with birth control? IVF is about getting pregnant and birth control is about preventing pregnancy, right? And aren't I aware that this is a book about birth control? Indeed, I am.

I'd like to make a case that two things are true. First, IVF and birth control are, in many ways, the same. Hear me out. They are both modern tools that help us build the family that we want. Sometimes these tools are successful; they help us have babies when we want them and to remain baby-free when we don't. (And in fact, as anyone who has gone through IVF can tell you, birth control is actually used during IVF treatments to regulate cycles, so these two modern tools are even more intertwined than you might think at first glance.)

And sometimes these tools fail us. Sometimes we want something, and even with these amazing modern tools, we don't get what we want. Failures can lead to broken hearts. Failures can make us rethink our goals and plans. Sometimes we find new joy and happiness in a pathway that wasn't what we thought we wanted.

The process of family building—whatever number of parents and children that means—is one that can take years. It can be an emotional rollercoaster; it can have the highest of highs and the lowest of lows.

What's the second way that IVF and birth control are the same? Like IVF, birth control is under threat. In fact, they are under threat for the very same reasons. Laws that can be interpreted to protect fertilized eggs not only impact IVF services but also birth control. And in the bigger picture, IVF and birth control both represent choice and progress for a broad range of people and families—a fact which attracts attention that is not always positive.

The fates of IVF and birth control are intertwined. The future of family building is like a cliff, and we are all standing on the edge.

Hanging in the Balance

In March 2018, Mississippi passed the Gestational Age Act, which banned abortion after fifteen weeks. The law provided exceptions for medical emergencies and severe fetal abnormality but no exceptions for rape or incest. On the day the law was passed, Mississippi's only abortion clinic, Jackson Women's Health Organization, filed a lawsuit to challenge the law's constitutionality. The suit was brought against state health officials, including Thomas E. Dobbs, a health officer with the Mississippi State Department of Health.

So started the long, legal battle to the Supreme Court. First, the US District Court for the Southern District of Mississippi ruled in favor of Jackson Women's Health Organization. The state of Mississippi appealed the decision. At the Fifth Circuit court, Judge Patrick Higginbotham upheld the district court's ruling: "In an unbroken line dating to *Roe v. Wade*," he said, "the Supreme Court's abortion cases have established (and affirmed, and re-affirmed) a woman's right to choose an abortion before viability."

Mississippi appealed the decision again, this time to the Supreme Court. In May 2022, someone—and we still don't know who—leaked a draft of a majority opinion written by Justice Samuel Alito. What many people feared was confirmed: the federal right to abortion was to be struck down after fifty years. When the *Dobbs v. Jackson Women's Health Organization* decision was formally released on June 24, 2022, *Roe v. Wade* was done.

Why does this matter for birth control? It matters for many reasons. In *Roe v. Wade*, the basis for the right to abortion was a "right to privacy," which prior Supreme Court cases had ruled was implied in the Constitution. Those prior Supreme Court cases? They were about birth control.

You see, there isn't actually a federal law guaranteeing an American citizen's right to privacy. Nor is there anything in the Constitution that guarantees us that right, either. The word privacy doesn't even show up in the Constitution. Our "right" to privacy has actually been bestowed upon us over time through a series of Supreme Court decisions which have ruled that regular citizens have a reasonable expectation that the government will give us some privacy to go about our everyday lives. And for decades, that right to privacy has been secured by the precedent set by those prior Supreme Court decisions.

In striking down *Roe*, the Supreme Court ruled that because the right to privacy wasn't explicitly stated in the Constitution, there wasn't a good enough case to keep *Roe*. When *Roe* was struck down, Justice Thomas argued in a concurring opinion that the Supreme Court should reconsider other cases that relied on the same principles as *Roe*. What other cases was he referring to? Cases that established the right to birth control. Suddenly, the right to birth control is not as secure as it had been.

Since *Roe* was overturned, twenty-one states—primarily in the Southeast—have banned abortion. Seven states ban abortion at some point during pregnancy (ranging from six to eighteen weeks). Fourteen states have banned it entirely. Many articles and books have successfully argued that access to abortion is a health care issue. Not having the ability to terminate a pregnancy puts lives in danger; it's as simple as that. Like birth control and IVF, abortion is an essential family building tool. But while abortion gets a lot of attention, birth control does not—which is why I'm making it the focus of this book.

And in some cases, these abortion bans can be misinterpreted as limiting not just abortion, but also birth control. In Missouri, for example, some people think that the total abortion ban applies from the moment the egg is fertilized. When the governor refused to say that the Missouri abortion ban would *not* apply to birth control methods, a major hospital in Missouri stopped providing Plan B (also known as the morning-after pill). They were worried that they would be charged with violating the law because of a common misunderstanding about how Plan B works.

Plan B is one type of "emergency contraception." Emergency contraception is often confused with medication abortion, but they are different. Emergency contraception does not end a pregnancy. Plan B prevents the body from releasing an egg ("ovulation") but does not prevent the egg from being fertilized or implanted.

It wasn't until after the Missouri Attorney General's office clarified that the abortion ban would not apply to Plan B that the hospital began offering it again.

The story that unfolded in Missouri is unfolding elsewhere, too. In 2020, Texas stopped paying for emergency contraception with public dollars. In 2021, Missouri voted to stop their public insurance program from covering emergency contraception (though ultimately the law didn't pass). In 2021, Idaho passed a law that prevented school-based health clinics from providing emergency contraception, except in cases of rape. And in 2023, Iowa stopped reimbursing for emergency contraception, *even for survivors of sexual assault.*

Like Plan B and other emergency contraception pills, IUDs (which stands for intrauterine devices) are also under threat. IUDs work primarily by preventing sperm from reaching an egg (to do this, IUDs make cervical mucus thicker and inhibit sperm movement). They work early in the process to stop a pregnancy from happening rather than disrupting an existing pregnancy. Yet, there is real concern that as states interpret abortion bans to apply from the moment of fertilization—as in Missouri and also Tennessee—and if people misinterpret how birth control methods work, the result will be that it will be harder to get birth control methods like the IUD and Plan B.

We are already seeing the effect of the abortion bans on birth control: fewer people are getting the birth control that they want. In 2024, researchers published a study of women eighteen to forty-four years of age living in four states: Arizona, Iowa, New Jersey, and Wisconsin. The study compared two time points, one before and one after *Roe v. Wade* was overturned. During that time, the researchers found a significant increase in women experiencing trouble with or delays in getting their preferred birth control. Young people were the most likely to experience trouble getting birth control. There was also a significant decrease in women receiving health care services related to birth control, including counseling and education about birth control.

Though it's impossible to say for sure how much the *Dobbs v. Jackson Women's Health Organization* decision caused these changes, the researchers go on to say, "As we continue to experience the fallout of the Dobbs decision on access to abortion, this research makes clear that many people are also experiencing worsening contraceptive care."

So where does that leave us? We're standing on the edge of that cliff. For a lot of people, the right to birth control has never been guaranteed. Still, for others, it's a right we may have taken for granted in the past. We shouldn't take it for granted any longer. Our ability to build families when and how we want is more at risk than ever before. There's never been a more important time to care about birth control—and to do something about it.

* * *

In the coming chapters, you'll come to understand why I think birth control gets so much *public* attention even if it is not a favorite topic of dinner conversation in our private homes (except for my house, where I can assure you it is *the* topic of dinner conversation). I'll hopefully convince you that birth control is not controversial, though it's sometimes made to seem that way.

You'll see why men don't share in the burden of using birth control, and whether that's ever going to change. You'll take a look at the dark parts of the not-so-distant history of birth control, and how important it is to use that history to make sure the mistakes of the past aren't repeated today. This might be hard to read if it is new information for you, but it is important.

Finally, I'll walk through the methods that are available today (information which you may or may not need, depending on where you are on your birth control journey), the many benefits of birth control that go beyond preventing pregnancy, and the impact of birth control on gender equality—driving improved health outcomes, increased education, and improved economic stability and advancement. Finally, I'll share a few steps that I hope you will be ready to take after you finish this book.

Maybe you are reading this book for you, or maybe you're reading it for your partner, daughter, sister, or friend. Whoever you are, my hope is that when you finish this book, you will have a greater appreciation for birth control. I hope that the information in these pages will help you make your own decisions about birth control. And I hope that this better understanding of birth control will spark your support for the idea that everyone, everywhere should have the right to make decisions that impact their families.

Remember

- **Birth control is universally used.** Most people are using birth control currently, and just about everyone has used birth control at some point in their lives.
- **The right to birth control is at risk.** The same "right to privacy" that was struck down when *Roe v. Wade* was overturned underpins the right to birth control.

1

In the Beginning

When Crocodile Poop Was Your Best Option for Birth Control

Legend has it that it was a warm summer day, and Persephone, Goddess of fertility, was out for a stroll admiring the flowers. Suddenly, the world split open beneath her feet. Out sprang Hades, God of the dead, who grabbed Persephone and sped her back to the underworld, where he held her as his prisoner. Persephone's disappearance devastated her mother, Demeter, who immediately abandoned all her goddess duties, causing mass drought and famine. As the drought spread, Zeus was compelled to try bringing Persephone back to the land of the living. Hades reluctantly consented to releasing Persephone, but before she exited the underworld forever, Hades handed her a pomegranate. Little did Persephone know, eating the pomegranate seeds would prevent her from being able to leave Hades' kingdom of the dead.

Alas, eat the seeds she did. Zeus was, understandably, angered by Hades' ploy. So, Zeus and Hades agreed to a compromise: Persephone would return to the land of the living but rejoin Hades as his wife for a third of the year, during which time the world would return to a cold, barren state. And each year, when Persephone leaves the underworld, she sparks new life to return as the Goddess of Spring.

The story of Persephone is often thought to be about the cycle of life, death, and rebirth. (And maybe also a critique of the patriarchy? How come neither Hades nor Zeus ever think to ask Persephone about where *she* wants to live, eh?) The pomegranate is seemingly a small detail to point out. Pomegranates show up in all sorts of stories, myths, and legends, and they have many different meanings. The seeds hidden by the smooth exterior have come to represent duality, being both individual and part of a whole. The fruit symbolizes immortality, eternity, and resurrection—the cyclical relationship between life and death. It symbolizes fertility and infertility, rebirth, and times of transition from being a part of something to a whole, such as going from childhood to parenthood.

Fun fact: pomegranates were, in the time of the Ancient Greeks, also frequently used as birth control. Full of contradictions, pomegranate seeds were understood to be fertility enhancing.[1] The emptied-out rind, on the other hand, was sometimes used as a barrier placed inside the vagina (for the record, this is not something I recommend trying).

One interpretation of this tale might be that Hades handing Persephone the pomegranate was less about desiring her company back in the underworld and more about exerting control over Persephone's body and reproduction. Was Hades trying to trick Persephone into becoming pregnant? It certainly wouldn't be the first or last time in history that this has happened.

The interpretation I prefer? (And please allow me some poetic license, here.) Persephone, being a goddess of agriculture in her own right, would have been fully aware of the many uses of pomegranates. She knew that after she ate the pomegranate, she would use the rind for her own purposes. When she took the pomegranate from Hades' hand, she also took control back for herself.

* * *

Humans have been curious about reproduction since the dawn of time. For almost as long as humans have been capable of thought, we've known there was a connection between sex and pregnancy, though we didn't fully understand the biology of reproduction until much later. Our ancestors' confusion about how exactly sex causes pregnancy was quite understandable. Pregnancy doesn't happen every time you have sex. Before people understood the ovulation cycle, it seemed like pregnancy happened randomly. In the earliest days, humans believed that divine intervention and the movements of the sun, moon, and stars played a role. (Even knowing the biological processes, I would venture that a lot of us—myself included—still see something of a miracle within the science of pregnancy.)

Another thing that made it hard to predict and really understand pregnancy was that it used to be impossible to see what was going on inside the body or at the microscopic level. Even though the human egg is the largest cell in the body, it's still only the size of the period at the end of this sentence. A sperm cell is about *one millionth* of the size of an egg, far too small to be seen with the naked eye. Before microscopes, humans had no idea how eggs and sperm worked—we literally couldn't see them!

The first microscope was invented around 1600, and not long after, scientists saw eggs and sperm for the first time. It was a major breakthrough in our understanding of human reproduction. Eggs and sperm were discovered separately, which kicked off a long debate about the relative importance of each. (Ah, how I wish I could have watched that debate unfold. I imagine two toddlers fighting over who is right. Eggs! No, Sperm! I'm right! No, I am!) The debate was settled in 1875 when a German scientist, Oscar Hertwig, observed a sea urchin egg fertilized under the lens of his microscope. As he watched, two distinct entities, egg and sperm, fused into each other. It turns out, we do need both. (The resigned parent to the fighting toddlers: "You are *both* right," before an eye-roll to the sky.)

Naturally, our ability to *prevent* pregnancy dramatically improved once we understood exactly how pregnancy was caused. But even before that happened, long before we knew about sperm and eggs, humans figured out how to avoid getting pregnant. Some of the methods used by our ancestors have proven to be legitimately effective. (Other methods . . . well . . . not so much.)

Your Wandering Uterus

Imagine for a minute that you're watching a scene unfold in the bedroom of an ancient Egyptian woman. She looks vaguely like Cleopatra. (Because, if we're being honest, I don't have much by way of imagination, and she is the only ancient Egyptian woman I know, and even that is a stretch because I really only know how she is portrayed in modern media. Anyway, I digress.) Her hair is black and shiny, hanging loose down her back. A light linen tunic hangs breezily from her bronzed arms. Kohl surrounds her dark eyes, drawing the attention of her partner to her face. She traces her fingers down the arm of her partner and makes eye contact in, you know, *that* knowing way. And just as things are really starting to heat up, she pauses and says to her partner seductively, "just hold that thought while I go get some crocodile dung."

It turns out that our friends, the ancient Egyptians, were excellent record keepers and documented all sorts of medicinal practices—birth control included. We know, for example, from the *Kahun Gynaecological Papyrus*, which dates back to about 1800 BC, that one recipe for birth control was to mix sour milk and crocodile poop into a paste. How appetizing! While the concoctions were nicely detailed for us, sometimes the instructions for use were less clear. Some modern readers think that the paste was placed into the vagina to cover the cervix. It's possible that the alkaline nature of the dung would have killed off sperm before they could fertilize the egg. However, it's probably more likely that the dung was burned, and the smoke fumes wafted near and around the vagina (a practice called "fumigation," recommended for many of the described prescriptions).

The *Kahun Gynaecological Papyrus* was one of two important pieces of writing that give us insight into the medical practices of ancient Egypt. The other is the *Ebers Papyrus*, which dates back to about 1500 BC. The *Ebers Papyrus* is a 110-page, 60-foot-long scroll describing hundreds of medical formulas and remedies. It's famous for its "treatise on the heart" that describes it as "the center of the blood supply with vessels attached for every member of the body" and contains such eerily beautiful explanations as, "When his heart is afflicted and has tasted sadness, behold his heart is closed in and darkness is in his body because of anger which is eating up his heart."

Apparently, the Egyptians held the heart in higher regard than the uterus. The uterus (also called the womb) is the pear-shaped organ in a woman's pelvis where a baby develops during pregnancy. Reading the *Kahun Papyrus* leads one to believe that the uterus is the root cause of most bodily complaints. Many prescriptions involve placing concoctions in, around, and near the problematic organ. Sometimes, mixtures were placed into the vagina (in the form of a "pessary" or ring). Other times, ingredients were burned near the woman so her body could absorb the wafted fumes. Some recipes called for simply spreading ingredients on top of the woman's stomach.

Donkey milk, honey, natron (a carbonate salt used for cleaning), fermented acacia leaves, and crocodile poop were just a few of the ingredients used. Today, we know that honey has some fertility properties if consumed; however, I think we can be sure there weren't any contraceptive benefits when it was "sprinkled over the womb," as suggested.

We also know the Egyptians used condoms, though this may have been more about preventing the spread of diseases than pregnancy prevention. Tutankhamun's tomb contained a condom made from linen, thoughtfully included for him to use in the afterlife.

Condoms and spermicides were also popular in the ancient empires of Greece and Rome. Aristotle recommended cedar oil, lead, and frankincense mixed with olive oil for spermicides. Greek physician Aetios suggested cedar resin and myrtle, lead, and wine in the vagina; he also suggested coating the penis with pomegranate, gallnut, and vinegar. King Minos of Crete was said to have used goat bladders as condoms to prevent disease.

In ancient times, women commonly consumed plants like vitex, pine, and pennyroyal to prevent pregnancy. It was typical for women to pass down their knowledge of plants to their daughters, sisters, and friends, and while documentation of the practices was mostly done by men who had the privilege of learning to write, it was in all likelihood women who were the original keepers of that knowledge. Today, we know that many of these ingredients do prevent pregnancy, though some, like pennyroyal, can be toxic in higher quantities.

Ancient Greeks and Romans also used the sap from a flower called silphium for birth control (as well as for other medicinal purposes—turns out the flower was a bit of a wonder drug). Grown only in Northern Africa, in a city in present-day Libya, people figured out that it was genuinely effective at preventing pregnancy. As such, it was in extremely high demand. Julius Caesar is said to have kept a stockpile of the plant in his treasury, as it was so valuable. Unfortunately, the demand for the flower became so high that it was overharvested to extinction by the fourth century.

Like the Egyptians, the ancient Greeks had some opinions about the uterus. They believed that the uterus was a separate entity from the body, and that wafting sweet odors in and around the vagina would bring about a pregnancy, and conversely, strategically placed foul odors could ward one off (ah, were it only that simple). They believed that the uterus could wander far enough that it would implant into the mind and cause a delirious, frenzied state (hence why hysteria and hysterectomy share the same origin, hystera, which means womb in Greek). Naturally, some practices to avoid pregnancy included spitting into a frog's mouth three times and wearing a leather pouch filled with cat's liver on one's left foot.

While the ancient Greeks didn't understand how pregnancy resulted, they—along with generations of people before them—had figured out that breastfeeding could effectively space pregnancies. Using breastfeeding (also called chestfeeding) as birth control is today known as the lactational amenorrhea method (LAM). The act of breastfeeding tells the body to stop releasing eggs and to stop having a period. LAM can be highly (98 percent) effective birth control if the breastfeeding person is not having a period, the baby is under six months, and the baby is being exclusively breastfed on demand both day and night. (There appears to be a biological response that only comes about when the baby physically suckles, so exclusive pumping is not thought to confer the same effects. Pacifier use is thought to reduce the pregnancy protection effect, too.)

The Natural Balance

Our knowledge of ancient birth control practices is largely dependent on cultures that placed a particular value on the written word. Another such culture with a penchant for writing things down was ancient India. The ancient Indian medical system, Ayurveda, dates back to more than 3,000 years ago. Written texts dating back to these ancient times document thousands of formulations for treating and preventing all sorts of diseases.

Among these were many specific prescriptions for birth control—powders, pastes, and other substances taken orally or applied before sex. Ayurveda texts make reference to *Kanji* (fermented drink), *Tandulodaka* (rice water), *Sarkara* (sugar candy), milk, honey, and eighty other plant-based concoctions for pregnancy prevention or termination. Some substances used in these prescriptions have been shown to help lower one's fertility. On the other hand, some prescriptions recommend using lead, mercury, and arsenic (all highly toxic substances), so maybe check before you take any recipe at face value. Still, the natural and holistic approach recommended in Ayurveda is compelling to many people who adhere to traditional methods today.

Over time, women in India and nearby countries, like Sri Lanka, have passed down their traditional knowledge of pregnancy prevention. Some women in this region recommend eating a papaya a day to someone wishing to prevent pregnancy. In fact, papaya contains an enzyme, papain, that interacts with the naturally produced hormone progesterone to prevent pregnancy. How about that for a super food?

Like the Indian Ayurveda, traditional Chinese medicine has been practiced for thousands of years. Physicians in ancient China were almost exclusively men. But the value placed on modesty for women made it challenging for men to treat women effectively. It was customary for women to need a male chaperone while being seen by a male doctor, and the doctor might question the chaperone instead of the patient. The doctor might not even see the woman or touch her directly.

One exception to this rule, however, was Tan Yunxian. Born in 1461 to a family of physicians, her grandparents saw her potential from a young age and engaged her in learning their medical practices. She wrote what is now considered to be the earliest known writing by a female doctor in China, *Miscellaneous Records of a Female Doctor*. Across her thirty-one case reports, she shared the traditional herbs prescribed, as well as her assessments and recommendations for patients seeking care for pregnancy, birth control, and pregnancy termination (as well as dozens of other acute and chronic conditions). Being a woman herself, Tan Yunxian primarily treated women and was able to provide them with a higher standard of care than what they were able to receive elsewhere.

Traditional Practices of Indigenous Peoples of Africa and the Americas

What is noteworthy when digging through the approaches to pregnancy prevention throughout history is that while the ingredients used in ancient communities varied across decades and places, at the same time there were some common birth control practices that evolved. Across most cultures, common methods of birth control have included not having sex during times of fertility (or "periodic abstinence"), withdrawal or the "pull out" method, and breastfeeding. These traditional methods require nothing beyond commitment from the parties involved. They are still commonly used today. About one in ten women across the world currently uses these traditional methods.

One of the many reasons that traditional methods became important was to space pregnancies. In lower-resource settings like low- and middle-income countries, pregnancies that are too close together have an increased risk of maternal and infant death. In higher-resource settings like the modern-day United States, the relationship between birth spacing and maternal and infant death becomes less strong. However, it still takes time for the body to heal after pregnancy, which is why the American College of Obstetricians and Gynecologists recommends waiting six months after one pregnancy ends before becoming pregnant again.

In communities all over Africa, women have long understood the importance of child spacing to infant and maternal health. Even when large families were encouraged, women may have been looked down upon when the spacing between children was viewed as too close. Postpartum abstinence and breastfeeding have commonly been used to help space children.

Other traditional birth control formulas were made from herbs, barks, and seeds. Because there was a lot of variation in the recipes, it has been hard to study the effectiveness of the formulas. But we do know that African women brought knowledge of traditional herbs and plants with them to the colonies when they were forced from their homes as enslaved people. Women who were enslaved applied their knowledge to prevent pregnancies that their owners forced upon them and to prevent having children who would be forced into slavery.

In the seventeenth and eighteenth centuries, indigenous women of the Americas understood that they could predict their fertility based on the consistency of the discharge that comes out of the vagina. (This is technically called "cervical mucus," and I'm honestly not sure whether that or "vaginal discharge" is a less appealing term.) They used that information to avoid sex if they were trying to prevent pregnancy. In the 1960s, Australian Drs. John and Evelyn Billings conducted research that scientifically proved what indigenous women had long understood. Vaginal discharge becomes clear and slippery (similar to raw egg whites) and can be stretched between two fingers immediately before and during ovulation. This is a natural indicator of fertility. If you are trying to prevent pregnancy, it's best to avoid sex on days when you or your partner is experiencing this type of discharge.

Understanding natural indicators of fertility has long been an effective way to prevent pregnancy. A typical menstrual cycle is twenty-six to thirty-two days long, and pregnancy is most likely during days eight to nineteen, during which time ovulation happens. So if someone is trying to avoid pregnancy, they can choose to avoid sex or use a different method on those days when pregnancy is more likely. Body temperature also increases slightly during ovulation. These "fertility awareness-based" methods of birth control are still very much used today. As of 2019, about one in five Americans had used them for birth control. These same indicators can also be used to help someone get pregnant by having sex around the time of ovulation when pregnancy is most likely.

Same S***, Different Millennium

So, what do we take away from the stories of our ancestors and their attempts to delay or prevent pregnancy? For one, women have been willing—or sometimes forced—to put themselves at extreme risk in order to have some control over reproduction. While in some cases we have since learned that ancient remedies were moderately effective birth control, a lot of the things that women ingested or inserted into their bodies were toxic, dangerous, and even deadly.

Why would women put themselves at such risk? Because the alternative was often worse. Women endured many pregnancies. In ancient Greece, women had six live births on average. And childbirth could be deadly. By some estimates, as many as one in three women in ancient times died in childbirth. Unsafe practices to terminate pregnancies also resulted in death and debilitation. It wasn't just a fear of their own death that led women to try to prevent pregnancy. Women had to endure the pain of watching their children die. For much of human history, about half of babies born didn't make it to their fifth birthday. Giving their existing children adequate resources was another reason people sought to prevent pregnancy.

While these risks are certainly lower today, they are not altogether gone. Women in the United States are much less likely to die due to pregnancy-related causes today than they were hundreds of years ago—but there are significant and troubling differences by race and ethnicity. Black women are three times and American Indian and Alaska Native (AIAN) women are two times more likely to experience a pregnancy-related death, respectively, compared to white women. The gap widens for women between the ages thirty and thirty-four, when Black and AIAN women in the United States are about four times more likely to have a pregnancy-related death.

Infant deaths are, fortunately, also much rarer today. But while the overall US infant mortality rate is 5.6 per 1,000 live births, the rate is almost double for non-Hispanic Black women, Native Hawaiian and other Pacific Islanders, and American Indians. These are not problems that have gone away.

Controlling reproduction has been a life-or-death situation for women across generations. Looking back over the birth control practices of ancient times, I appreciate the safe and effective methods we have today; albeit it has been a long road to get there with many setbacks along the way. The methods we have today are more effective at pregnancy prevention than we've ever had before. But while much has changed with regard to safety and efficacy of birth control over the past several thousand years, there's a striking amount that is the same.

People across cultures and times evolved to use birth control that works fundamentally the same as methods we have today. For millennia, we have had condoms to block sperm and "spermicides" made from substances placed into the vagina. Orally ingested plants and herbs were the predecessors to the modern-day pill. Yes, over time, we have learned a lot about the human body, which has helped us develop better birth control methods. And in other ways, we've been simply building a better mousetrap since the dawn of time.

Finally, as we look back on the history of birth control, it's worth returning to this question of how we have the information that we do have—and therefore what information is missing. The knowledge of delaying and avoiding pregnancy has been knowledge centralized in the experiences of women. It was women who took risks, trying different concoctions or materials and testing them out with their own bodies. It was women who told their daughters and sisters about their experiences, sharing what they had learned and drawing on the experiences of others to refine recipes and guidance.

Yet, documentation has historically largely been practiced by men, especially men who were physicians or clergy. While Hippocrates, known to many as the "father of medicine," documented many herbal recipes for birth control (including one recipe for a ring filled with mutton fat inserted into the vagina), he likely gets credit for recipes that were passed down through generations of women before him.

We're lucky that many folk remedies continue to be passed down by women across generations, so that we may continue to better understand them. Who is to say what our ancestors knew but didn't, couldn't, or wouldn't write down?

Missing Links

When I was first interested in getting birth control, it didn't occur to me to ask anyone I knew about it. Ask my friends? How embarrassing. Ask my mother?! Mortifying! The internet was new enough that the idea of going to Dr. Google didn't cross my mind either. I went in for my doctor's appointment essentially knowing nothing about birth control. I didn't know what my options were, how they worked, how long they lasted. I just knew that I didn't know how to swallow pills and hoped there was an option other than the well-known pill. (And meanwhile, I practiced swallowing pills. How could I swallow food and not pills? I will never understand.)

Birth control used to be something that women learned about through the mutual sharing of recipes, fertility indicators, and traditional practices. And while it is common to learn about birth control from a friend or family member, we no longer share and hold knowledge about birth control in the same way that our ancestors did. In many ways, that's a good thing. We rely on trained professionals for accurate information. On the other hand, there is some basic information about birth control that we simply don't have.

Consider the following questions from the Contraceptive Knowledge Assessment. Try to answer each question.

Select only ONE answer for each question.

1. How long can sperm stay alive in a woman's body?
   a. 1–3 hours
   b. 24 hours
   c. 3–5 days
   d. 7–10 days
   e. I don't know
2. Which one is NOT a benefit of hormonal birth control?
   a. Improvement of diabetes
   b. Improvement of acne
   c. Reduction in menstrual cramps and bleeding problems like anemia
   d. Decreased risk of ovarian and uterine cancer
   e. I don't know
3. What is the main way that birth control pills work?
   a. It prevents the ovary from releasing the egg (ovulation)
   b. It prevents sperm from entering the uterus
   c. It prevents the fertilized egg from implanting in the uterus
   d. It prevents the embryo from growing past a certain size
   e. I don't know
4. How long after a woman stops using birth control can she become pregnant?
   a. Immediately
   b. 1 month
   c. 3 months
   d. 6 months
   e. I don't know
5. If you forget to take one birth control pill and remember the next day, what should you do?
   a. Throw the missed pill away and then continue the following day from where you left off
   b. Take the rest of the week's pills at once and then start the placebo ("reminder") week
   c. Take two pills then continue
   d. Throw the missed pill away and wait 1 month to start a new pack
   e. I don't know
6. A doctor places an IUD (intrauterine device) in what part of the body?
   a. Fallopian tube
   b. Uterus
   c. Cervix
   d. Vagina
   e. I don't know
7. Which choice is FALSE about IUDs?
   a. Women of all ages may get an IUD
   b. Women who have never had a baby may get an IUD
   c. Women can have an IUD put in right after having a baby or having an abortion
   d. Women cannot get an IUD if they have ever had a sexually transmitted disease (STD)
   e. I don't know
8. A doctor places the birth control implant in what part of the body?
   a. Thigh
   b. Vagina
   c. Arm
   d. Buttock
   e. I don't know

9. How soon after sex must the "morning after-pill" (or Plan B) be used to be effective?
   a. 1 h
   b. 24 h
   c. 5 days
   d. 20 days
   e. I don't know

10. How can you get the emergency contraceptive pill called Plan B (or "the morning-after pill")?
    a. If under age 18, you cannot get it, even with a prescription
    b. If under age 21, you must have your parent go with you to the doctor for a prescription
    c. All women must have a prescription, no matter her age
    d. You can buy it at the pharmacy, without a prescription, no matter what age
    e. I don't know

Answer Key: 1:C, 2: A, 3: A, 4: A, 5:C, 6: B, 7:D, 8:C, 9:C, 10:D
Note: The full Contraceptive Knowledge Assessment is twenty-five questions. I've included a subset of questions here for simplicity.
Source: Haynes, Meagan Campol, Nessa Ryan, Mona Saleh, Abigail Ford Winkel, and Veronica Ades. "Contraceptive Knowledge Assessment: Validity and Reliability of a Novel Contraceptive Research Tool." *Contraception* 95, no. 2 (February 1, 2017): 190–97. https://doi.org/10.1016/j.contraception.2016.09.002.

How did you do? If you found yourself scratching your head, randomly selecting an answer, and crossing your fingers you weren't wildly off base, you are not alone. When the researchers who developed this assessment tested it with 102 reproductive-age men and women, on average people got 36 percent of the questions right. When researchers repeated the study with medical students, they did a bit better, answering 78 percent of questions correctly. As someone who is *not* a medical professional, I find it comforting to know that health care providers do know this stuff better than most of us. But at the same time, it reinforces just how much knowledge about birth control is centralized within a small subset of the population.

It's not just that we're missing facts about birth control. It's that we *feel* like we don't have the information we need to make informed choices for ourselves. Only three in ten women report feeling like they received all the information they needed before they chose their method of birth control, and this is lower among Asian/Pacific Islander, Hispanic, and Black women.

Many women do not know, for example, that insurance plans are, in most circumstances, required to pay the full cost of birth control and have been required to do this since 2012, thanks to the Affordable Care Act.[2] At a minimum, plans have to cover at least one of each type of birth control method for free (so for example, a plan might cover one brand of IUD but not all of them).

Yet one in four women pays some money out of pocket for birth control. Some women are doing so knowingly. For example, they want a certain brand of contraception that is not covered by their insurance plan (even though insurance should cover a method if it is recommended by a provider), or they use an out-of-network provider or pharmacy. But 50 percent of women do not know why birth control is costing them money. If you're paying out of pocket for birth control, you might not need to. Or if you have been under the impression that getting on birth control is expensive, you might think again.

Another case in point: One in four women either haven't heard of emergency contraceptive pills, like Plan B, or don't know that they can be bought over the counter, despite the fact that this has been true for more than fifteen years. Among women who have heard of emergency contraceptive pills, 31 percent don't know where they can get them. (In many cases, they can be purchased at a drugstore or grocery store, but not all stores carry them, and they can be especially hard to get in rural areas.)

Remember

- **For as long as people have been having sex, they have used birth control.** Even before we fully understood pregnancy, humans capably derived ways to prevent it.
- **Today's birth control methods work in ways that are similar to ancient methods, but they are much safer and more effective.** Women have gone to great lengths to prevent pregnancy and in doing so cultivated a deep knowledge of birth control practices. Not all of the methods they used were safe, but pregnancy was often even less desirable.
- **We deserve to have the information we need about birth control.** Without accurate information about birth control, how can we expect to make informed decisions that impact our health, lives, and families?

2

Strange Bedfellows

The Complicated History of Birth Control, Religion, and Politics

In 1276, a man by the name of Peter of Spain wrote a book with extensive, meticulously organized, and detailed information about dozens of ways to prevent and terminate pregnancy. *Thesaurus Pauperum* (*Treasury of Medicines for the Poor*) was a well-circulated handbook designed for ordinary people, particularly people who could not afford a doctor. This man, with a background in medicine, theology, and physics, would later become Pope John XXI. That's right: A Pope led the effort to distribute information about birth control to the masses—surprising given the Catholic Church's strong anti-contraception stance.

The conventional wisdom is that birth control and religion are battlefield rivals. But in truth, the story is more complicated. Nearly all of the major religions have a great deal of openness to pregnancy prevention. And that's fortunate. Because people of all religions have sought ways to prevent pregnancy for, well, forever.

Are Birth Control and Religion Really Worst Enemies?

Let's start with a basic fact. People of all religions have sex. Procreation is a religious fundamental. Think: go forth and multiply. How many begets and begots are there in the Bible? It's funny (to me, at least) that sex is both taboo and also *the* building block of religion. One can't exactly blame the forebears of major religions for their emphasis on sex; in order to continue to survive as a species, we need future generations, and the same is true of religious communities. Children are needed to secure our fate as a community. So, naturally then, procreation (sex) is hallowed, sacred, aspirational.

What else is common to major religions? Preventing pregnancy. Primarily to manage family size and preserve the health and wellbeing of religious practitioners. For example, it's said that Buddha considered family size a personal choice and advocated that choosing *not* to have children could help alleviate suffering—the ultimate goal. Destroying life is prohibited in Buddhism, but birth control is generally seen as preventing the creation of life and therefore acceptable. Ancient Hindu texts also suggest an openness to birth control. *The Kama Sutra*, written by Vatsyayana in the early fourth century, is one way that we know sex has been considered a natural part of life among Hindu cultures for centuries. Ancient Ayurvedic texts describe multiple ways to prevent pregnancy.

Even within other major religions—like Islam, Judaism, and Christianity—there is, perhaps, a surprising amount of openness to pregnancy prevention. Obviously no ancient religious texts say anything about modern birth control; birth control is simultaneously as old as time and extremely new. And the most conservative of readings can, of course, lead someone to conclude that only the methods explicitly mentioned in religious texts are acceptable.

But many texts also provide some insight into *why* preventing pregnancy is acceptable, like in order to preserve the health of mothers and existing children and to ensure that existing children have the resources and care that they need to thrive. Applying that insight to modern contexts has led many religious scholars to interpret birth control as morally acceptable.

Religious texts nearly exclusively talk about preventing pregnancy in the context of heterosexual, married couples who are assumed to desire families. Obviously, this is a very narrow view. In today's world, plenty of people who are not heterosexual or married use birth control for a whole range of reasons. Not everyone is or wants to be a parent. When ancient religious texts were written, cultural norms around sex in and outside marriage looked very different. Many religious scholars accept that when the world changes, so can our interpretations of religious texts. (Of course, not everyone comes to the same conclusion.)

Let's look at Judaism, for example. In the Torah, Gen. 1:28 says, "And God said unto them, Be fruitful, and multiply, and replenish the earth, and subdue it." Some understand this to mean that humans, and really men in particular, have a divine duty to procreate. (Sometimes this is interpreted to mean that any birth control that destroys sperm is not acceptable.) But at the same time, the Talmud, the primary Jewish text on religious law and theology, makes space for birth control. The Talmud recommends using a sponge soaked in vinegar (called mokh) to prevent pregnancy in order to keep mothers and babies healthy (e.g., one time that birth control is recommended is while a mother is breastfeeding so she doesn't get pregnant and have to stop nursing prematurely.) What does this all mean? Within the Jewish tradition, many religious scholars and practitioners agree that sometimes birth control is warranted, especially if it means preserving health.

In Islam, the prophet Muhammad is said to have endorsed the withdrawal method both to protect the health of the mother and to promote the financial security of families. The Qur'an encourages mothers to breastfeed infants for two years, which, by the way, so does the American Academy of Pediatrics. The Qur'an's recommendation of prolonged breastfeeding is meant to space out births and keep moms and babies healthy.

Muslim-majority countries like Pakistan, Bangladesh, Indonesia, Iran, Turkey, and Tunisia have established government-funded programs that have been providing birth control for several decades. While uptake of modern birth control methods has been lower in Muslim-majority countries compared to other countries, these methods are becoming more accepted. This has led to a dramatic drop in the number of babies women deliver. In 1995, women who lived in all forty-nine Muslim-majority countries had an average of 4.3 children; by 2015, this had fallen to 2.9.

Which Brings Us to Christianity

The Catholic Church is the only major religious authority—Christian or otherwise—that says birth control conflicts with their faith. The story of Onan in Genesis is often cited as the basis for this stance. Onan refused to impregnate his recently widowed sister-in-law, electing to instead "spill his seed on the ground." God grew mad at Onan for failing to perform his duty of giving his deceased brother a child. So, naturally, God killed him for it.

What's the message here? Try to prevent pregnancy, and God will smite you. At least, that's how some Christian authorities over the years have interpreted it. In the second century, the theologian Clement of Alexandria argued that sex could only be justified for reproduction. But we really have to thank theologian and philosopher Saint Augustine, who two hundred years later argued in his book *Marriage and Concupiscence*[1] against any form of birth control— including natural family planning methods—a text that influenced official Christian thinking on the topic for *over 1,000 years*. (While Saint Augustine and I disagree on basically everything, I've got to hand it to the guy that it's impressive to be just *so* convincing to shape a millennium of thought. In the era of social media, is *anyone* today capable of such a lasting impact?)

When in the 1500s Protestantism and Anglicanism evolved from the Catholic Church, their views on contraception were aligned (which is to say, collectively opposed). But following the Industrial Revolution and in response to mounting social pressure, these denominations loosened their stance. Prior to 1930, authorities advised married couples trying to avoid pregnancy to not have sex during times when the woman was most likely to get pregnant ("periodic abstinence"). Understandably, many parishioners didn't like this policy. So in 1930, the Anglican Church issued an official statement in support of birth control (within the context of marriage). Other Protestant denominations followed suit soon after.

The Catholic Church, on the other hand, doubled down on their opposition to birth control. In 1930, Pope Pius XI wrote in *Casti Connubii* that the use of any methods of birth control except periodic abstinence amounted to "grave sin." When the birth control pill came onto the market thirty years later, a number of theologians, thought leaders, and Catholic parishioners appealed to the Church to rethink their stance. They argued that having sex during infertile periods was the same whether the hormones that regulated those infertile periods were produced by the body or in a lab.

Those appeals fell on deaf ears. In 1968, Pope Paul VI released *Humanae Vitae (Of Human Life)* which reaffirmed the strict prohibition on birth control and stated that "The Church, nevertheless, in urging men to the observance of the precepts of the natural law, which it interprets by its constant doctrine, teaches that each and every marital act must of necessity retain its intrinsic relationship to the procreation of human life." Translation: sex is for procreation, not for pleasure.

Does It Even Matter?

So, because the Pope forbids birth control, Catholic people refuse to use it, right? Actually, that's not the case at all. It turns out American Catholic women are just as likely to use birth control as women of other faiths. Across all religious affiliations, nearly all American women have ever used a method of birth control *other than* natural family planning methods. (Just 1 percent of Americans who have a religious affiliation have relied exclusively on natural family planning methods.) In 2017:

- 99.0 percent of Catholics had used birth control methods like the pill, IUDs, or condoms; as did
- 99.6 percent of women with no religious affiliation;
- 99.4 percent of mainline Protestants;
- 99.3 percent of evangelical Protestants; and
- 95.7 percent of people with other religious affiliations.

Looking at current birth control use, about 25 percent of Catholic women report using short-term hormonal birth control methods like the pill. Another 25 percent have been sterilized, and another 15 percent are using long-term hormonal birth control methods like the IUD.

At any given time, about one in six women are not using birth control. Of those women, just 4 percent say it's because of religious reasons. That means out of every thousand American women, just seven are foregoing birth control because of their religion. That's not to say that the women who choose to use birth control don't care about their religion. I would venture that many of these women feel very connected to their faith, and some might even feel conflicted by their choice to use birth control. But at the end of the day, women decide that the benefits outweigh the drawbacks, and they choose to use birth control. In other words, religion doesn't really play the major role in our decision to use or not use birth control that we have been led to believe.

In contrast to official Catholic Church teachings, most American Catholics don't subscribe to the idea that birth control is immoral, either. Just 5 percent of Americans think using birth control is morally *unacceptable*. This is about the same when you look at all Christian denominations (4 percent) and only slightly lower than among Catholics (8 percent).[2] In 2013, nearly three quarters of Catholics agreed that their church should permit birth control. Birth control really *isn't* controversial after all.

(And by the way, the story is similar when we look at abortion. While more than half of Catholics think abortion is morally wrong, the same proportion believe it should be legal in all or most cases. A majority of people who get an abortion have a religious affiliation, and one quarter of people who get an abortion report they are Catholic. This is in spite of the Catholic Church's firm anti-abortion stance.)

So how did the Catholic Church become entrenched in their opposition to birth control? To understand that is to understand the fear, greed, and anxiety of men who saw their livelihoods threatened and lashed out in response.

Witchcraft and Medieval Times

When our dear friend Peter of Spain, later Pope John XXI, published his *Treasury of Medicines for the Poor,* he drew on knowledge that had been passed down over hundreds of years by healers who were predominantly women. Though these women lacked formal medical training (which let's face it, at the time wasn't all that great anyway), they effectively gathered practices and understanding of the medicinal properties of plants, herbs, and other substances. They refined their remedies and shared their knowledge with their mothers, sisters, friends, and neighbors. While the medical establishment largely ignored or misunderstood the health care needs of women, women healers did not.

But between the fourteenth and seventeenth centuries, women healers became the target of clergymen and formally trained physicians who wanted to secure their power. Seeking to elevate their own credibility, these men launched a campaign to frame women healers as witches. It was both a power grab and just another example in history when women's reproduction was viewed as something to control. There were widespread labor shortages because the Black Death (bubonic plague) had wiped out as much as half of Europe's population in the mid-1300s. Since women healers provided reproductive health care, eliminating them effectively forced population growth.

Even while healers were persecuted and discredited, many women continued to seek out their services. But over time carrying the knowledge of healing practices became increasingly dangerous.

Women who had the knowledge to care for and treat reproductive health concerns, like pregnancy prevention, became more and more fearful about being accused of witchcraft or heresy. So it's no surprise that knowledge about how herbs and plants could be used for birth control began to slowly disappear in Europe after the thirteenth century. Some of it was undoubtedly lost, and some of it was co-opted by the formal medical and religious establishments.

The Victorian Era: Let's NOT Talk about Sex

Unfortunately the medical and religious establishments weren't always the best stewards of information about birth control. Through the 1800s religious authorities, along with religiously motivated political authorities, tried to scare people by warning them about the moral and physical dangers of birth control and pregnancy termination. Despite that, between 1835 and 1935, the number of children the average American woman gave birth to over the course of her lifetime went from 7.0 to 2.1 (similar to what it is today). The United States went from having one of the highest to one of the lowest birth rates in the Western world. Did couples in the Victorian era stop having sex? Nope. But they did start to use birth control that was increasingly easy to get, accepted, and effective.

Sex was not something people spoke about in public during the famously repressed era. But privately, preventing pregnancy was on everyone's mind. As one 1888 editorial in the *Journal of the American Medical Association* put it, "We do not exaggerate: everyone that knows anything of American society in cities (at least) knows that there are very few married people that do not or have not discussed methods of preventing conception, and the majority of physicians will have no difficulty in remembering instances in which they have been consulted on this subject." Everyone, it seemed, was talking about birth control.

In the early half of the 1800s, the common methods of birth control were withdrawal and periodic abstinence. The Voluntary Motherhood Movement was a particularly strong advocate for periodic abstinence. Among the movement's spokespeople were feminists Elizabeth Cady Stanton and Susan B. Anthony. They urged married couples to go without sex to control family size.

Unfortunately for its staunch advocates, abstinence can be hard to adhere to. And when you fail to adhere to it, well, it doesn't work great. So couples turned to other forms of birth control on the market: suppositories and pessaries (removable devices placed into the vagina that physically block the cervix), douching with acidic solutions, and antiseptics used as spermicides. Advertisers used code words that were poorly kept secrets, referring to such devices as "feminine hygiene," "female tonic," and the entirely unhelpful "Mother's friend."

On the market were pills or loose herbs, which could be prepared in tea or dissolved into alcohol, that induced menstruation. Ingredients varied wildly—this was before the time of ingredient lists on the back of the bottle—but included things like pennyroyal, rue, hellebore, mistletoe, savin, foxglove, and Queen Anne's lace (many of the same herbs that had been used for centuries to the same effect). Wintergreen or spearmint might have been mixed in to make the remedies more palatable.

At the time, people erroneously thought that douching would prevent pregnancy. Early douches were syringes that you aimed into the vagina to "clean it." Douching syringes were frequently used with cleaning solutions. The practice of douching remained popular for decades; in the 1930s through the 1960s, one could purchase douching kits from drug and grocery stores, and Lysol disinfectant was a top-selling "feminine hygiene" product. We now know that not only is douching ineffective at preventing pregnancy, it can be extremely harmful. Douching alters the healthy state of the vagina, and can inflame, irritate, and even burn the vagina and cervix.

Condoms were also available at the time. Through the early 1800s, condoms were primarily made from sheep, calf, or goat intestines (how lovely!). But that changed in 1837 when Charles Goodyear and Thomas Hancock discovered that rubber became stable and elastic if mixed with sulfur and subjected to high heat—a process called vulcanization. Vulcanized rubber revolutionized condom production, but even rubber condoms had some issues. Early rubber condoms only covered the tip of the penis and, by some accounts, weren't particularly comfortable. They could be bought from brothel and tavern owners, which didn't help their reputation either. The stigma around condoms was apparent from the nicknames people used for them. Americans called condoms French letters, the French referred to them as redingotes Anglaises (English riding coats) and capotes Anglaises (English capes), and across Europe they were known as "American tips."

By 1860, condoms were being produced at a larger scale, which made them more affordable. But even at $1, compared to an average weekly pay of $14, condoms were still expensive (unlike modern condoms, however, they were washable and reusable). Over time, as production processes improved and condoms became easier to produce, the demand for them soared, and the term "rubber" took on a whole new meaning.

While modern birth control methods like condoms became more mainstream during the 1800s, so did information about birth control become more readily available. Not everyone was happy about this. And nothing spurs people to action like fear that the world is changing around them faster than they can handle.

Religion and Politics Converge

By the mid-1800s, several states had started to legislate "obscene materials." The New England and mid-Atlantic states, with their puritanical roots, were among the most aggressive in fighting against obscenity. What kind of "obscene" materials were lawmakers trying to protect citizens from? One physician, Charles Knowlton, was fined and sentenced to three months hard labor in Massachusetts for writing a plain-language book about sex and anatomy. In Pennsylvania, another author, Frederick Hollick, was sued twice on obscenity charges because he included anatomically correct drawings of reproductive systems.

The first of these so-called "obscenity prosecutions" occurred in 1815. The Commonwealth of Pennsylvania charged Jesse Sharpless for showing a painting of "a man in an obscene, impudent, and indecent posture with a woman." The controversial painting was hung in the privacy of Sharpless's own home! The Pennsylvania Supreme Court ruled that seeing such an image could corrupt the minds of young people by "inflaming their passions" and found Sharpless guilty of obscenity. This happened even though there wasn't even a law against obscenity in Pennsylvania at the time.

The ruling was a victory for proponents of the Second Great Awakening. Their mission was to integrate evangelical Christian beliefs into American laws and politics. Their platform included banning alcohol, blasphemy, "sins of the flesh," and (gasp) Sunday mail delivery.

Part of what drove followers of the Second Great Awakening to push for a "moral reckoning" was that society was becoming more liberal, especially when it came to sex. One of the places this was most apparent was on the battlefield. Soldiers had condoms and porn shipped to where they were stationed. Sexual misconduct and sexually transmitted diseases ran rampant. Sex was such a part of life for soldiers fighting in the Civil War that the Union army provided government-sanctioned prostitution in cities like Nashville and Memphis. These cities had programs for licensed prostitutes that included registration, medical exams, and medical treatment (and the programs did work to reduce the spread of sexually transmitted diseases.)

Seeing what he viewed as soldiers' moral failures spurred one Anthony Comstock into action. Born in 1844 in New Canaan, Connecticut, Comstock was raised by a devout Congregationalist mother who instilled in her son a fierce religious fervor. Comstock was raised to believe that complete and total abstinence from all impure thoughts and behaviors would lead him to righteousness. As a soldier for the Union army, he campaigned against the use of tobacco, alcohol, gambling, and atheism. He joined the Christian Commission, which was created by the Young Men's Christian Association (YMCA) to send ministers to preach to soldiers about the importance of morals.

After the war, Comstock moved to New York City. He was immediately appalled by the commercial sex industry, the freely available porn and erotica, as well as the widespread use of birth control and abortion services. He went on a personal crusade to hold tradespeople accountable to an 1865 obscenity law that criminalized sending any "obscene book, pamphlet, picture, print, or other publication" through the mail. He helped police raid and arrest booksellers and other merchants by spying and feeding information to police. Comstock attracted the attention of a number of wealthy benefactors who shared in Comstock's distress about the state of morality in the city. They established the New York Society for the Suppression of Vice, which hired Comstock as a full-time employee.

Comstock decided that in order to achieve real change, he needed to go bigger. Individual state actions against obscenity were no longer sufficient; he wanted a federal law. So in 1872, Comstock traveled to Washington and successfully lobbied Congress to pass the *Act for the Suppression of Trade in, and Circulation of, Obscene Literatures and Articles of Immoral Use*—which he drafted himself. The law was signed on March 3, 1873 by President Ulysses Grant. Now known as the "Comstock Act," the law prohibited people from mailing any items deemed "obscene, lewd, or lascivious," which specifically included items used for birth control.

The law also made it illegal to send any *writing* about the banned items—in advertisements, *but also even in personal, sealed letters*. Individuals who violated the Comstock Act could be fined up to $2,000 and sentenced to five years of hard labor. For his leadership in passing the law, Comstock was appointed a special agent for the post office. That position gave him the authority to identify people violating the law and arrange their arrests. At the time, the United States was the only Western country to criminalize birth control at the national level.

Buoyed by Comstock's success at the federal level, twenty-four states followed the Comstock Act by enacting laws that prohibited the sale and distribution of birth control. The most restrictive state was Connecticut, where even the use of birth control was prohibited. According to Connecticut law, married couples who used birth control even while in their own homes could be arrested and given a prison sentence of up to a year. While the Connecticut law wasn't easy to enforce, just having the law on the books impeded people from getting birth control or information about it.

It took decades for the major parts of the Comstock Act to be struck down, and that was only achieved through the concerted efforts of some brave birth control advocates. One such advocate was

Dr. Hannah Stone, a physician at a birth control clinic. In 1936, Dr. Stone, with the help of fellow birth control advocate Margaret Sanger, ordered a new type of diaphragm from a Japanese physician in Tokyo. They anticipated that the package would be seized and confiscated when it arrived in the United States They actually *wanted* the package to be confiscated to kick off a legal challenge to the Comstock law. In a US Circuit Court of Appeals decision, *United States v. One Package of Japanese Pessaries,* the court ruled that physicians could now legally mail birth control devices and distribute information about birth control for medical purposes throughout the country. The following year the American Medical Association supported birth control for the first time.

That case signaled an increasing level of support for birth control in the general public. Such public support continued to grow, especially with the release of the first birth control pill in 1960. But even though physicians were by then permitted to prescribe birth control, state laws still prevented people from getting it. Then in 1965, the Supreme Court struck down the restrictive Connecticut law that made birth control illegal even in private homes. Estelle Griswold was the executive director of the Planned Parenthood League of Connecticut. Together with her colleague Lee Buxton, a physician and professor at Yale Medical School, Griswold was charged with providing married couples information about and prescriptions for birth control. In *Griswold v. Connecticut,* the Supreme Court ruled, by a vote of 7–2, that the Connecticut law banning birth control violated the "right to marital privacy." The right to birth control was established.

Well, to clarify—the right to birth control was established *for married people.* Seven years after the *Griswold* decision, reproductive rights advocate William Baird was charged with a felony for distributing condoms and spermicide to unmarried students at Boston University. He would distribute them after delivering lectures on birth control and population control topics. He knew that birth control could only legally be distributed by a physician and to married people. He expected, even hoped for, the opportunity to challenge these outdated requirements. His case made it to the Supreme Court, and in *Eisenstadt v. Baird*, the Court ruled in Baird's favor. The Court stated that the Constitution guaranteed equal protection to unmarried and married people, and that if married people could get birth control—as established by the decision in *Griswold v. Connecticut*—then unmarried people had the right to it too.

To recap: It wasn't until 1972 that unmarried people had the right to get birth control. In that same year, Idris Elba, Dwayne Johnson, and Gwyneth Paltrow were born. The NASA Space Shuttle program launched. In 1972 my mother was a freshman and my father a sophomore in high school. Nixon was president . . . for the time being (we'll come back to him in just a minute). This is not ancient history by any means. This is the history of our lifetimes.

And it's not even really *history*. History implies that this is in the past. The story of Comstock and the right to birth control is not in the past. It was the "right to privacy" in *Griswold v. Connecticut* that established a married person's right to birth control, *and* then provided the foundation for the *Roe* decision. When *Roe*—and the right to privacy—was struck down, it had the effect of pulling a leg off of the stool on which the right to birth control sits. When the Supreme Court said that the right to privacy, the basis of *Roe*, was an insufficient argument to hold up *Roe*, the cases before it were suddenly called into question. These cases that secure the right to birth control are like dominoes, and the first one has fallen(Figure 2.1).

The Comstock law hasn't gone away either. Technically, it's still the law of the land, as it's never been repealed. It was the *Roe*, *Griswold*,

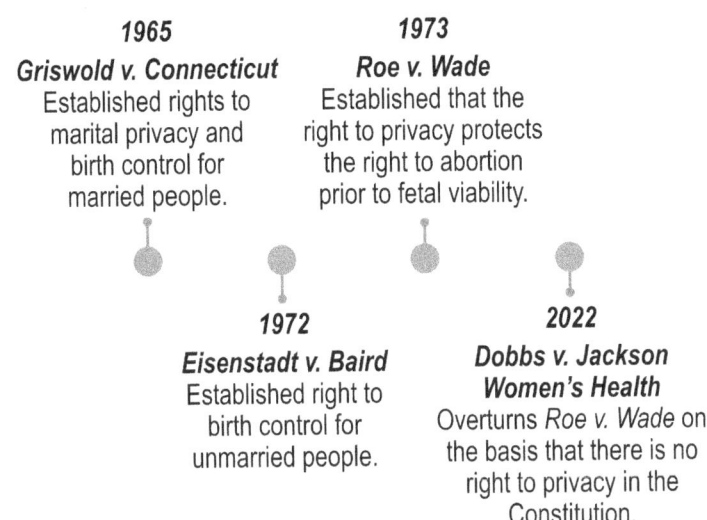

Figure 2.1 *A timeline of major Supreme Court decisions impacting reproductive health and rights.*

and *Eisenstadt* Supreme Court decisions that rendered the law moot. But as the decisions in those cases have become less secure—and repealed in the case of *Roe*—the reemergence of the Comstock laws is more likely. Already, we have seen some conservative thought leaders and lawmakers propose using the Comstock Act to ban mailing medication abortion or even supplies used in surgical abortion. This could have the effect of a national abortion ban, without having to pass any new federal legislation. When it comes to birth control, the *Griswold* and *Eisenstadt* cases stand. For now.

Remember

- **Nearly all major religions are open to using birth control.** Protecting the health of mothers and babies has long been a reason for religions to endorse pregnancy prevention.
- **People of all religions use birth control.** A very small portion of people do not use birth control for religious reasons.
- **The crusade against "obscene" materials landed birth control in hot water in the 1800s.** The law passed by Anthony Comstock has not gone away and is being threatened as a way to ban supplies used for abortion.

3

From Obscene to Ostracized

Population Control and the Origins of "Family Planning"

Something else was shaping opinions about birth control in the mid-1900s: exponential population growth. The world population grew from one billion in 1804 to two billion in 1928. Then it took just thirty-two years to reach three billion in 1960. As the world approached that major milestone, there was growing angst about humanity's rapid consumption of natural resources. (Sound familiar?)[1]

American politicians were especially concerned with worldwide population growth. In 1959, President Eisenhower's *Committee to Study the United States Military Assistance Program* (known as the Draper Committee) recommended that the United States support programs that distributed birth control and related health care services—coined "family planning programs"—to deal with the perceived problem of rapid population growth. Providing financial support for birth control in other countries was seen as a long-term investment in international economic development.

In 1967, under President Lyndon B. Johnson, Congress authorized funds to support family planning programs in other countries (notably before they did so within the United States). A policy popular with both parties, the bill to provide funding for family planning programs abroad was sponsored by twelve Democrats and six Republicans.

While the United States' support for international family planning programs has helped millions of people choose if, when, and under what circumstances they want to be a parent, the funding came with not-so-subtle pressure by the US government to shape *which* communities had fewer children. The original motivation for public funding for birth control was to urge poor families to have fewer children. This was true for both international family planning programs and US-based family planning programs.

A Political Pendulum

With international aid for family planning secure, politicians turned their attention to establishing a family planning program that would provide birth control for Americans. Title X (read as "Ten") of the Public Health Service Act created the first—and, still to this day, the only—federal program dedicated to providing birth control for people who want it. There was strong bipartisan support for domestic family planning funding. In the House of Representatives, it sailed through with a vote of 298 to 32, a feat which now seems inconceivable. The bill was cosponsored by two Democrats, Sen. Joseph Tydings (D-MD) and Rep. James Scheuer (D-NY), and

Republican Representative and future US president George Herbert Walker Bush of Texas, who said in 1969, "If family planning is anything, it is a public health matter."

In 1970, President Nixon signed the Title X legislation. The year before, he had declared that "No American woman should be denied access to family planning assistance because of her economic condition." Signing Title X into law fulfilled that promise.

But as Nixon prepared for his 1972 reelection campaign, he abruptly reversed his stance. In the two years since he first enacted the Title X family planning program, his political advisers convinced him that he could divide the Democratic Party—convincing Catholic Democrats to vote Republican—by withdrawing his support for birth control. Getting Catholics to vote Republican would help him secure a victory.

Why might previously Democratic-voting Catholics flip to vote Republican? Because over the preceding decade, while support for birth control was increasing, abortion laws were also becoming more liberal. Over the 1960s, several states implemented laws that legalized abortion (at least in certain cases). This scared the Vatican and, in part, prompted Pope Paul VI to write *Humanae Vitae* in which he advocated vehemently against both abortion and birth control. So, in an effort to sway Catholic voters to turn out for him, Nixon, who just two years earlier had championed the Title X program, now argued against its renewal.

One of the bills that legalized abortion—contributing to the political and religious realignment happening over at President Nixon's office—was passed by none other than Ronald Reagan during his time as governor of California. In 1967, Reagan signed a law that legalized abortion in cases of rape, incest, and in situations where the mother's mental or physical health was in danger. Reagan was a reluctant supporter of the bill. He ultimately signed it, but would later regret the decision and publicly announce that signing the law had been a mistake.

Reagan was outwardly deeply informed by his faith when it came to abortion. His mother, Nelle, was a devout member of the Disciples of Christ, and she is often credited with influencing Reagan's commitment to living a religious life. Reagan frequently attended services at Bel-Air Presbyterian Church and considered himself a "born-again Christian."

He may have also been haunted by the death of his second daughter, Christine, who was born premature and who passed away just a day after she was born in 1947. While Reagan didn't speak about losing a child in public, and never connected it to his views on abortion, it's hard to imagine how such a devastating event could *not* impact his beliefs—especially beliefs related to family building and raising children. Reagan's daughter, Patti, would later argue that the violent language common to the anti-abortion movement—such as the killing of unborn children—triggered her father's trauma of losing a child, perhaps unknowingly strengthening his stance on the issue.

Influenced by his own faith and advisers who shared his beliefs, Reagan advanced not only an anti-abortion but also anti-birth control agenda. It is, in large part, thanks to him that the two issues of abortion and birth control have become so politically intertwined that they have since been impossible to disentangle. Reagan moved the federal Title X family planning program from the Health Services Administration (now the Health Resources and Services Administration) to the Office of Population Affairs in the Office of the Assistant Secretary of Health. This was more than paper pushing. It enabled his office to have more direct oversight of the program by a political appointee. His administration encouraged federal programs to emphasize abstinence, adoption counseling, infertility counseling, and nonhormonal contraception (the "natural family planning" methods) instead of comprehensive sex education, unbiased pregnancy options counseling, and counseling about the full range of birth control methods.

Reagan withdrew all funding for the United Nations Population Fund that advocates for—and delivers—sexual and reproductive health services, including birth control around the world. He withdrew funds from organizations if they performed abortions, provided counseling about or referrals for abortions, or lobbied to make abortion legal or more available in their own countries— even if these activities were performed with other funding *not* from the US government (a policy known as the "Gag Rule"). Reagan's administration attempted to apply a similar gag rule to reproductive health care providers in the United States who receive funding from the Title X program, but a legal challenge prevented the policy from going into effect.

Nearly four decades later, the Trump administration would pick up this same policy and succeed in implementing it within the Title X program. Then, two years later the Biden administration repealed the policy. And back-and-forth volleying is basically how things have gone since the Nixon administration. Funding for international family planning programs and the extent to which reproductive health providers working in publicly funded clinics can *talk* about abortion (never in the history of the Title X program have those federal funds been able to pay directly for abortion) have become issues that swing like a pendulum every time there is a new political party in the White House.

The pendulum swinging might, on the surface seem inconvenient, irritating, tiring. And it is certainly all of those things. It is frustrating for reproductive health providers to constantly change practices, especially when they are asked to do things that conflict with the recommendations of medical professional organizations. But the effect of rapidly changing policies is worse than being merely exhausting. When funding is withheld from family planning programs, both internationally and domestically, the very real result is that fewer people have access to the reproductive health care they need, including birth control.

Changing Times for Religion in America

The role of religion in the lives of Americans looks very different today than it did during Reagan's administration. The share of Americans who say religion is "very important" in their lives fell from 70 percent in 1965 to 51 percent in 2018. In 2016, nearly eight out of every ten Americans agreed religion was losing its influence on American life.

As religion plays a less central role, we are looking elsewhere for information and guidance to inform our values. Where previously we may have looked to religion, we now rely on other sources of information—the media, the internet, our social networks—to inform our beliefs. Religions have historically relied on families to transfer expectations and values across generations. As we rely more on information that comes from outside of the family, our approach to answering questions about sex, intimacy, and relationships has changed.

Understandably, people respond differently to this shift. Some people fear that greater availability of birth control and information about sex, sexuality, and relationships will encourage behaviors they find unacceptable. The data tells a different story: talking about sex, birth control, STIs, and healthy relationships doesn't increase the chances that people, even young people, will have sex. A huge analysis that combined sixty-six different studies showed that people who receive comprehensive sex education are less likely to be currently sexually active, they have fewer sex partners, and they have less unprotected sex and tend to make more use of condoms and other types of birth control compared to people who don't.

On the flip side, abstinence-only sex education has consistently been shown to actually raise the risk of unintended pregnancy. States with laws that stress abstinence-only education have the highest rates of babies born to teens, while states with laws that mention abstinence as part of a discussion of comprehensive sex education (or that don't mention abstinence in state laws at all) have the lowest teen birth rates.

In reality, nearly all parents, across the political spectrum, agree that sex education in high school should cover a broad range of topics. Most parents agree that high schoolers should get information about STIs (98 percent), healthy relationships (96 percent), abstinence (96 percent), puberty (95 percent), and birth control (94 percent).

Unfortunately, some politicians play to people's fears by pitting birth control as somehow against "traditional family values." This conflicts with most major religions that almost universally accept that pregnancy prevention is a part of ensuring the health and well-being of people and families. It also conflicts with what most Americans think; just 5 percent of Americans believe birth control is morally unacceptable. And the fact that 99 percent of American women have used birth control is perhaps the best indication of how truly uncontroversial we understand birth control to be. When politicians oppose birth control, it contradicts what most actual Americans believe and how we act. As is true for so many things, when it comes to birth control, we agree on far more than we disagree.

Remember

- **Birth control became a political issue, thanks to a few highly committed individuals.** Anthony Comstock and Ronald Reagan were motivated by faith. Richard Nixon was motivated by winning (at least the guy is consistent!).
- **Funding for birth control initially enjoyed bipartisan support,** but more recently, when political parties changed in the White House, so did support for reproductive health services like birth control.
- The political pendulum when it comes to birth control stands in contrast to the fact that the **vast majority of people find birth control both morally and personally acceptable**.

4

It Takes Two

Why We Don't Have a Birth Control Pill for Men—and How Close We Are to Getting It

Sometimes I think about all of the many hours that I have spent going to and from the pharmacy to pick up a birth control prescription, or to and from the clinic to meet with a provider about birth control. Hours upon hours of my life have been spent getting birth control, and that doesn't even begin to include the many, many hours spent *thinking* about birth control. Is it working right? Is this random symptom I am experiencing a side effect of birth control? Should I be changing my birth control to something better?

Then I think about how many hours of my husband's life he has spent getting birth control. It's zero hours. Even when I generously add in the time he's spent thinking about birth control . . . it still basically rounds to zero hours.

Now to be clear, I don't think men are villains in this story, shirking their responsibility. The methods that are available for men are simply not that great. The world of birth control is designed pretty much exclusively for women. And men and women actually agree that men should play a bigger role in pregnancy prevention than they currently do. So, will we ever live in a world where both men and women share the burden of preventing pregnancy?

The birth control pill for women has been around for a (relatively) long time; it was approved by the US Food and Drug Administration (FDA) in 1960. But what may be surprising is that it was not long after, starting in the 1970s, that researchers began trials on hormonal birth control methods for men. Many methods for men have proven effective, and some methods are even in the final stages of development before they can become widely available. That's exciting news! But if the research into these methods has been going on for more than *five whole decades*, why are we still living in a world where women continue to carry most of the burden for birth control?

Where Are We Now?

And carry the burden we do. In 2019, the United Nations reported that male-centered birth control accounted for only 28 percent of worldwide birth control use (mostly condoms, but also withdrawal and vasectomy). In other words, just about one in four men are helping to prevent pregnancy.

Research into reliable birth control for men didn't just start in the 1970s. For millennia, people have been devising strategies to reduce fertility in men. The Greeks hypothesized that heating up the testicles might reduce fertility. It turns out they were onto something. The scrotum tends to be 1–2 degrees cooler than the body and works as a natural air conditioning system for sperm. Modern studies show that warming the testicles a few degrees can reduce sperm count, though it's not entirely clear why. In 1956, Swiss physician Marthe Voegli found that men who sat in a hot bath for forty-five minutes a day for three weeks were protected against pregnancy for six months. It's a wonder why that hasn't caught on more. A prescription for long, hot baths? Sign me up, please!

If you *were* getting excited about luxuriating in the bath, I hate to have to tell you that medical professionals do not endorse soaking in a tub for birth control. But the desire to find reliable methods is understandable. There are really only three (!) birth control methods for men: withdrawal, condoms, and vasectomy. Only condoms and vasectomy are approved by the FDA, which regulates drugs and medical devices. Compare that to the more than fifteen options that are available to women (and within most options there tend to be several brands with varying levels of hormones that women can try). The birth control options for men are both limited and imperfect.

Withdrawal is an age-old practice. Remember the story of Onan in the Bible? People have been pulling out and "spilling their seeds" for thousands of years. Do we even need to review the drawbacks associated with the withdrawal method? For one, it's challenging to do it right every single time. And for this reason, it's not particularly effective; about one in five couples using withdrawal will get pregnant each year.

Condoms, as we have seen, have also been around for thousands of years. Early condoms were made from animal intestines or linen. In the mid-1800s, the discovery of the rubber vulcanization process made condoms easier to produce. Such was the dawn of the modern condom era. In 1920, latex (rubber suspended in water) was invented. Latex condoms were even easier to produce and had a longer shelf life than the original rubber condoms. Consumers also appreciated that latex condoms were stronger and thinner. Condom sales really took off from there. By 1931, condom manufacturers were producing more than 1.4 million condoms *per day*. By the 1960s, over 40 percent of Americans relied on condoms for birth control.

When used perfectly, condoms can be very effective. Maybe 2–3 percent of couples would get pregnant using condoms after a year of using them perfectly. But the reality is that few people use birth control perfectly. So it's more helpful to look at "typical use" effectiveness—in other words, how well a birth control method works in real life when used by real people. In the case of condoms, that number looks very different: 15 percent of couples who use condoms *actually* become pregnant in any given year. Condoms are still the only method for preventing STIs (besides abstinence).

There have been some recent efforts to innovate condoms. In 2013, the Bill & Melinda Gates Foundation paid companies to come up with new and improved condoms. They provided $100,000 for initial innovation grants, as well as the chance to win $1,000,000 to bring a new product to market. A number of good ideas were generated, but no new products made it to market. One of the more exciting options was the Origami Condom, which folded like an accordion and claimed to enhance sexual pleasure. But you won't find the Origami Condom in your local drugstore. That is in part because the FDA has special standards for companies trying to bring new medical devices to market, and so far, no companies have been able to surmount these standards.

Beyond condoms, another option for men is to get a vasectomy. About 500,000 American men get a vasectomy every year. About 50 million, or 5 percent of American men of reproductive age (eighteen to forty-five) have had a vasectomy. Men who are white, who were born in the United States, and who have higher levels of education and income are most likely to get vasectomies. The odds of having had a vasectomy also increase with age and the number of biological children.

The overwhelming benefit of vasectomy is effectiveness. About 1 in 1,000 couples using vasectomy will become pregnant each year, one of the highest effectiveness levels of modern birth control. A vasectomy is considered permanent. Although it can be reversed, there are risks associated, and no guarantee that a reversal will be successful. Getting a vasectomy is relatively quick and easy, and it's associated with very few complications.

The first vasectomies were performed in the late 1800s. At first, eugenicists forced vasectomies upon men whom they deemed unfit to reproduce. The first reported vasectomy in the United States was carried out by Chicago-based surgeon A. J. Ochsner in 1897, who argued in his paper "Surgical treatment of habitual criminals" that vasectomy could be used to slow "racial degeneration." In 1902, a surgeon at the Indiana Reformatory reported he had sterilized forty-two inmates to prevent them from producing future criminals. (We'll look more closely at the misuse of sterilization procedures in just a bit.) It was around the time of the Second World War that men started to choose to get vasectomies for birth control.

Why Don't We Have Better Options for Men?

Condoms are a barrier method, which means they prevent sperm from reaching an egg and fertilizing it. Vasectomy is a surgical procedure to cut and seal off the vas deferens (the tubes that carry sperm from the testicles), so no sperm leave the body. In exploring new birth control methods, researchers are continuing to look at ways to prevent sperm from leaving the body or from reaching an egg to fertilize. But these aren't the only opportunities to interrupt biological pathways to prevent pregnancy.

For example, we could stop sperm from being created altogether. A perfect birth control method would lead to azoospermia which, despite what it sounds like, is not an animal park competing with Magic Kingdom for your kids' attention. Azoospermia means semen that's sperm-free. There are about 100 million sperm cells released during a typical ejaculation, so achieving complete azoospermia is unlikely. This is one reason why developing effective birth control alternatives for men is challenging. It's logistically much simpler to interrupt the production of one or two eggs per month produced by women than it is to inhibit the millions of sperm found in semen.

But we don't have to eliminate 100 percent of sperm to be effective birth control. Instead, the more realistic goal is less than one million sperm per mL of semen, a concentration shown to be 99 percent effective at preventing pregnancy. One challenge is that it takes some time for sperm to develop after they are created in the body, so a method that prevents sperm from being created wouldn't be effective right away. It would take two to three months to clear out the pipeline of existing sperm. Over the past several decades, there have been several hormonal and nonhormonal products—delivered as injections, pills, implants—tested in men that reduced sperm levels to varying degrees.

Reducing sperm's mobility—in effect, paralyzing the sperm so they can't reach an egg—is another way that birth control for men might work. In 2023, researchers injected mice with a mixture that made their sperm stop moving. This gave researchers hope that the mixture could someday be adapted for humans for the same effect.

Who Experiences Side Effects and Risks?

Researchers have hypothesized, observed, and tested dozens of birth control products that attempt to disrupt one or more of these processes. So why have none come to market? One reason is that our threshold for side effects and risks has gotten much higher over the past five decades.

When the original birth control pill for women was developed in the late 1950s, there were no formal standards for clinical trials (the research process which tests whether drugs or devices are safe and effective for people). The testing of the birth control pill in women who lived in Puerto Rico is considered highly unethical according to today's standards. The women weren't told that they were participating in a clinical trial, nor that the pill was experimental. When they complained of serious side effects (the original dose of the pill was much higher than it is today), their concerns were dismissed. Three women died during the trial, and there was no follow-up to exclude a link between the deaths and the pill. The lack of formal clinical standards trials put people, especially low-income people and people of color, at extreme risk.

Following the Puerto Rico pill trials, the FDA approved the birth control pill for women in 1960. In 1964, several doctors were charged with medical crimes committed in Nazi Germany at the Nuremberg Trials. In response, the World Medical Association came out with new ethical standards for clinical research referred to as the Declaration of Helsinki: "Because it is essential that the results of laboratory experiments be applied to human beings to further scientific knowledge and to help suffering humanity."

Among the basic principles established in the Declaration of Helsinki is that the potential benefits of any research must outweigh the risks to people participating in it. The Declaration says, "When the risks [to people participating in the study] are found to outweigh the potential benefits or when there is conclusive proof of definitive outcomes, physicians must assess whether to continue, modify or immediately stop the study."

Assessing the risks of men taking or not taking birth control is tricky. Since they don't get pregnant, they aren't at risk for any rare but serious complications related to pregnancy termination, carrying a pregnancy to term, or delivery. When men take birth control and pregnancy is prevented, it's women who experience the "benefit" of reducing their risk of pregnancy-related outcomes. According to the ethics of clinical research, it's not fair to ask men to endure the risks of taking birth control—side effects and rare but serious consequences associated with taking birth control—if they don't experience the benefits associated with pregnancy prevention.

Back in the 1970s, researchers discovered that a combination of testosterone and progestin (the same hormone used in birth control pills for women) resulted in a highly effective birth control pill for men: only five pregnancies took place over the equivalent of 180 years of taking the pill. However, there were side effects. Men taking the pill experienced mood changes, acne, oily skin, and weight gain. Women who have taken hormonal birth control will look at those side effects and find them quite familiar. Yet, some trials were stopped because the balance of risks and benefits was not as clear for men as it would be for women testing new birth control.

Of course, this is a flawed way to measure benefits and risks associated with taking or not taking birth control. Placing the burden of risks associated with pregnancy solely on women fails to acknowledge the role that men play in pregnancy. And while women might experience the physical consequences of pregnancy, men experience pregnancy in their own ways. Regardless of gender, there are emotional, financial, and logistical consequences of pregnancy. Accepting that the risks associated with pregnancy are shared would raise the threshold for what side effects are acceptable.

Bringing New Products to Market Is Challenging (as It Should Be)

The FDA's approval process can be long, challenging, and expensive. You've probably heard this before. It still bears mentioning just how rigorous the process is, especially because it hasn't always been this way.

A new medical device or drug starts as an idea, but to refine that idea, researchers undertake literature reviews, lab experiments, and computer simulations to get to a point where there is something specific the device or drug can target.

In preclinical development, researchers conduct testing in vitro (in cells) and in animals. They assess safety, toxicity, and side effects. They develop an understanding of how the body will react. They use all of that information to refine and optimize the product. It can take several years (even decades) to conduct this preclinical trial testing, and that alone can be millions of dollars.

Only if preclinical testing shows that the product is safe and effective do researchers move on from preclinical development to testing it with humans. Human clinical trials begin with a small cohort of healthy patients to test side effects (stage I), before moving to larger and larger groups of study participants in stages II and III. At each stage, researchers collect more information on side effects, safety, and efficacy. The clinical trials process can take several years and tens of millions of dollars to complete.

Only about one in five drugs that reach stage II clinical trials will move on to stage III. Only a select few make it out of stage III trials and are then designated for regulatory approval. When seeking regulatory approval, the manufacturer will submit all the data they collected during the prior stages to the FDA. The FDA rigorously reviews all the data, evaluates risks and benefits, and provides input on appropriate labeling. Just one in three drugs that make it through stage III trials ultimately clear regulatory approval.

Getting approval of drugs and devices is a necessarily rigorous process with intense regulatory oversight. We've seen what happens when manufacturers take shortcuts in the name of making a profit. This happened when the Dalkon Shield came onto the market in 1971. The developers advertised it as a superior, more effective, and easier-to-use IUD relative to the dozens of other IUDs on the market at the time. By 1974, 2.2 million American women were using the shield. Not long after it came out, however, research showed that the developers' claims of safety and effectiveness were overblown. The device had a 5 percent failure rate and a 6 percent expulsion rate—far higher than was originally advertised.

More importantly—and devastatingly—the Dalkon Shield was linked to pelvic inflammatory disease, uterine perforations, sterility, spontaneous septic abortions, and at least four deaths. Women who became pregnant while using the shield had serious life-threatening problems. There was a major design flaw: the IUD string was made of a material that carried unhealthy bacteria into the uterus. Although the device manufacturers knew about these problems by 1972, it took them another two years to issue a recall. Later, a class action lawsuit against the manufacturers would send them into bankruptcy, with $2.5 billion paid out to over 170,000 women in more than eighty countries who were harmed by the Dalkon Shield.

This catastrophe raised the alarm on the need for oversight of medical devices, which, at the time, weren't as rigorously evaluated as drugs. Congress passed the Medical Device Amendments in 1976, which assigned regulatory authority for medical devices to the FDA, created a risk classification system for devices, and required post-market monitoring and reporting of medical devices. Today, drug and device developers are required to collect data on effectiveness and side effects even after approval.

Where Do We Go Next?

All told, it can take as much as a billion dollars to bring a new drug or medical device to market. Usually, these immense costs are shouldered by large pharmaceutical companies, which stand to make a profit. However, in the case of birth control for men, it's not pharmaceutical companies driving research and development. The primary funders of research into birth control methods for men are the US government and mission-driven research organizations like the Population Council and the Male Contraceptive Initiative. Pharmaceutical companies abandoned the male-centered birth control market because they aren't convinced that men would actually *use* birth control.

The data on that question, however, is quite promising. Several studies have asked men this very question, including one online survey of 1,500 men between eighteen and forty-four living in the United States sponsored by the Male Contraceptive Initiative in 2019. They found that 80 percent of men say they feel sole or shared responsibility for avoiding pregnancy. Among men trying to prevent pregnancy, 81 percent were interested in new forms of birth control for men. From these results, the study authors estimate there are 13.7 million American men who are likely to use birth control.

But would women trust men to take birth control? This is often raised as a concern, but the data suggests that women think men are trustworthy partners. In a study of nearly 2,000 women living in Scotland, China, and South Africa, 98 percent of women said they would trust their partner to take a birth control pill. In a systematic review including thirty-two studies, between 42 percent and 94 percent of women said they would be willing to rely on a male-centered method of birth control.

To me, the question isn't about trust; it's about fairness. I've been taking birth control since I was sixteen. I've spent more of my life on birth control than not. I don't even really remember the person I was before birth control. My husband? Not so much. And while I don't mind taking birth control, I do find it irritating that we don't have to care equally about it. Would I stop taking birth control if my husband did? Probably not. I'm a control freak and, besides, why would I want to get my period after so many years without it? But I *would* appreciate the fairness of us both having to work to maintain the family size that we want.

So, many men say they would try birth control. Many women say they would trust men to take birth control. The future world where men and women share the birth control burden seems plausible. As we look to this hopefully not-so-far-away world, what birth control methods are men most likely to be using?

There are two birth control methods that are relatively close to coming to the market. The first is an injection of a nonhormonal gel-like compound into the tubes that carry sperm (vas deferens) through a minimally invasive, outpatient procedure using local anesthesia. The compound blocks sperm from traveling through the vas deferens without affecting sensation or ejaculation. Similar in concept to the "set it and forget it" IUD for women, this method lasts for years. And like the IUD, it's reversible; the compound can be dissolved when someone no longer wants it there. There are a few versions of the compound in development. RISUG—or reversible inhibition of sperm under guidance—has been shown to be 99 percent effective for up to ten years; it is in late-stage human trials in India. The other, ADAM™, lasts for two years and began human trials in 2022.

The other promising option is a hormonal gel, NES/T, that is applied daily to the shoulder blades. NES/T is made up of two active ingredients: nestorone® and testosterone. Nestorone® lowers sperm production to less than one million sperm per mL—the magic number that prevents pregnancy. Testosterone is added to keep blood testosterone at normal levels in order to maintain sex drive and function. The two active ingredients in NES/T are used in other drugs and are known to be safe and effective. NES/T is reversible, with sperm levels returning to prior levels about four months after stopping. In 2024, NES/T was in phase II clinical trials.

But we are still years away from seeing either the injectable compound or gel for the skin. A common refrain among researchers and advocates is that we have been ten years away from better birth control for men for the last fifty years. It can be hard to maintain a sense of optimism with how long it has taken us to get to this point, seemingly with nothing to show for it. But there *is* a lot happening behind the scenes, and we've never been closer to a world of shared responsibility for birth control than we are today.

And while we wait, we have a large menu of modern birth control options for women—the first, and still most popular, is the pill. And the story of two determined, unapologetic, and complicated women who got us the pill is one I think you should know.

Remember

- **Currently the only methods available for men are condoms, vasectomy, and withdrawal.** The options are limited, and all of these have some serious drawbacks.
- **Men say they would use birth control.** Women are interested in this too—and trust that men can be good partners in pregnancy prevention.
- **The two methods for men that are closest to prime time are an injectable, nonhormonal compound that could last years, and a daily hormonal gel.** We are still a few years away from seeing either of these methods.

5

The Magic Pill

How Two Women Changed the World Forever

When someone mentions "the Pill," you know exactly what they are talking about. Think about that. There are thousands of oral medications out there in the world. But only one is so well known that it is simply "the Pill." For more than four decades, the birth control pill has been the most prescribed medicine in the world.[1] More than seven in ten American women who have ever had sex have used the pill, and across the world, more than 150 million are currently using it to prevent pregnancy.

A Tale of Two Women Part 1: Margaret Sanger

The birth control pill was the lifelong crusade of one, Margaret Sanger. Born Margaret Louisa Higgins in 1879 in Corning, New York, Sanger was the sixth of eleven children. Growing up poor, she was profoundly shaped by the traumatic experience of losing her mother when she was nineteen. Sanger's mother died at the age of fifty of tuberculosis, but from her daughter's perspective, the true cause of death was the physical toll of *eighteen* pregnancies. Her mother endured eleven childbirths and seven miscarriages. Sanger blamed her father for causing these pregnancies, and ultimately, her mother's death.

Losing her mother propelled Sanger toward nursing. She attended Claverack College and completed her studies at White Plains Hospital in 1902. That same year, she married William Sanger, an architect, and they moved to Hastings-on-Hudson. They had three children. When in 1910 a fire destroyed their home, the Sangers decided to move to New York City.

Sanger got involved in a number of Progressive causes. She joined the Women's Committee of the New York Chapter of the Socialist Party and participated in efforts to advance women's suffrage and women's labor rights. She made friends with activists and intellectuals like Max Eastman, Upton Sinclair, and Emma Goldman. Her advocacy work also led her to Katharine Dexter McCormick, a fellow activist committed to the causes of women, who would change the trajectory of the birth control pill a few years later.

Sanger put her degree to work as a visiting nurse on the Lower East Side. She traveled to the homes of low-income and immigrant women, where she observed the toll that undesired pregnancies took. She cared for women recovering from complications of abortions. She cared for women who were malnourished themselves, struggling to afford food for their children. She cared for women who were visibly emotionally and physically exhausted from multiple pregnancies and caring for children. Sanger's patients reminded her of her own mother.

Women asked Sanger for advice about how to prevent pregnancy. But she had few options to offer them. Women could track their menstrual cycles and avoid sex during fertile days, but that required the cooperation of their partners. There were rubber condoms, but they cost money. Plus, women didn't always feel like they could ask their partners to wear them. The 1920s would bring cervical caps and diaphragms, barrier methods that prevent sperm from reaching the egg, but these required a visit to a doctor to be fitted and were paid for out of pocket. And further complicating matters, before Comstock had set his sights on passing a federal law, he successfully advocated for a New York State law that banned the trade and distribution of "articles of indecent or immoral use," which included birth control.

Angered by the suffering she witnessed—and frustrated by the lack of support women had when it came to avoiding pregnancy—Sanger decided that enough was enough. She would devote her energy to helping women choose if and when to become pregnant.

She started by trying to get better information out to women. She published *The Woman Rebel* in 1914 that advocated for "birth control," a term she coined. She was charged with violating the Comstock laws and fled to England to avoid arrest. Sanger returned from Europe to stand trial, only to be shattered by the death of her five-year-old daughter. Prosecutors dropped the charges against Sanger because public support for her was too strong.

That wasn't the last time Sanger was arrested. In 1915, she was indicted for mailing a package of diaphragms. In 1916, she, her sister Ethel, and an interpreter they worked with were arrested for opening a birth control clinic in Brownsville, Brooklyn. Sanger spent thirty days in jail that, to the dismay of her detractors, attracted the attention of the media and helped energize new supporters to her cause. "I see immense advantages in being gagged," she said in 1929. "It silences me but it makes millions of others talk about me and the cause in which I live."

For the next two decades, Sanger advocated fiercely for safe and effective birth control. In 1921, she founded the American Birth Control League, which solicited support for birth control from the medical community and the public. (The American Birth Control League would later become the Planned Parenthood Federation of America in 1942, for which Sanger was named honorary chairman.) She formed the National Committee on Federal Legislation for Birth Control to lobby Congress to allow physicians to prescribe birth control methods like diaphragms, which ultimately became legal in 1936 through the Supreme Court ruling in *United States v. One Package*. In 1927, she organized the first World Population Conference in Geneva.

But Sanger was a complicated figure and not without fault. Her passion for ending suffering caused by unintended pregnancies and a concern for rapid population growth blurred into a troubling overlap with eugenicists, who envisioned a world where "undesirable" people were prohibited from having children. Her work to bring birth control to Black communities—done in collaboration with Black leaders like W. E. B. Du Bois—when viewed in the context of her affiliation with the eugenics movement, is upsetting. She publicly proclaimed that "Birth control is nothing more or less than the facilitation of the process of weeding out the unfit [and] of preventing the birth of defectives." Her association with eugenics is a dark cloud that hangs over her legacy.

Problematic as she was, Sanger's work also heralded an era of increased freedom, autonomy, and progress for women. A few months before she died in 1966, Sanger witnessed the legalization of birth control for married couples in *Griswold v. Connecticut*. And while she wouldn't live to see it, the right to birth control would be extended to people regardless of marital status seven years later. Sanger's efforts pushed the field forward in incredible ways, even while much more remained to be done.

A Tale of Two Women Part 2: Katharine McCormick

Not too long after Sanger began her work as a visiting nurse on the Lower East Side, she began dreaming of a "magic pill" that would give women the power to prevent pregnancy. In the 1920s, the only birth control products that women could truly control were cervical caps and diaphragms. Though Sanger championed the diaphragm—she and her husband provided the funding for what became the first diaphragm manufacturing company in the United States—she understood its drawbacks. While more effective than periodic abstinence or condoms, a diaphragm could be expensive and required a doctor's visit to be fitted; both made obtaining one challenging for women. Sanger illegally imported diaphragms from Europe (where they were not illegal) and provided them to patients, sometimes even fitting women herself when she couldn't find a doctor to work with her, at least until she was shut down for breaking the law.

So while Sanger pushed legal boundaries with the goal of dismantling the Comstock laws that prevented people from getting birth control, she also wished for an easy-to-use, affordable, and effective method that women would *want* to use and could control themselves.

But Sanger was never content to simply wish for things. She made them happen. And in this case, she needed her longtime friend and collaborator McCormick to help. Sanger and McCormick met in 1917 when Sanger was delivering a lecture about birth control in

Boston. McCormick was moved by Sanger's passion, courage, and perseverance. McCormick shared Sanger's interest in women's health and rights, and the two struck up a conversation. They stayed in touch and became good friends. McCormick even helped smuggle illegal diaphragms into the United States for Sanger's birth control clinic.

Sanger and McCormick were set on the idea of developing a birth control pill. In 1953, they approached Dr. Gregory Pincus, an expert in human reproduction, and convinced him to join the project. Pincus had attended Cornell University and quickly made a name for himself in the field of biology. He was known for his innovative research. In 1931, he successfully used in vitro fertilization in rabbits, a feat that put him well ahead of his time. The public response was not as positive, however, and he was portrayed as a Dr. Frankenstein-type scientist conducting disturbing research in his laboratory. His career tanked. Without other prospects, he and a friend started the Worcester Foundation for Experimental Biology that focused on applied research. Though the work was satisfying, the foundation struggled financially, and Pincus served as the lab's janitor in order to save them money.

Rather than approach established university-affiliated research programs, Sanger and McCormick gravitated toward the little upstart foundation with a lot to prove. It was a mutually beneficial partnership: Pincus got an opportunity to conduct the innovative research he loved; Sanger and McCormick got a qualified scientist with no competing priorities and a shared interest in pushing boundaries. Pincus and his colleague Dr. Min-Chueh Chang, a specialist in fertilization in mammals, knew they were up to the task. Pincus had read a study that showed progesterone could suppress ovulation and decided to explore it further in his lab. Within just a few months, the pair proved that repeated injections of progesterone successfully stopped ovulation in animal testing.

On the other side of the world, chemist Russell Marker discovered that generations of Mexican women had been eating a wild yam called the Barbasco root, or cabeza de negro, for birth control. He extracted from the yams what would ultimately become a synthetic form of progesterone. Contributing this finding to the research literature was a critical step that would make a progesterone-based birth control pill a possibility.

To do their research, Pincus and Chang needed money. And that is where McCormick came in. McCormick was born into a well-known Chicago family in 1875. Her family prized education, and in an unusual move for the time, McCormick's father encouraged her to obtain a college education. She was the second woman to graduate from the Massachusetts Institute of Technology, with a major in biology.

She married Stanley McCormick, a wealthy heir to a large agricultural company fortune, after college. Just two years later, she was devastated when Stanley was diagnosed with schizophrenia. His health quickly declined. Concerned about the risk of passing the illness down, the couple chose not to have children, an experience that likely drew her closer to the cause of supporting women to choose when, or even if, they wanted to have children at all. She donated money to the suffrage movement and mental health research.

Stanley died in 1947, and his fortune of $15 million passed to McCormick. She began to generously support the birth control cause, so when Sanger pitched the idea of a birth control pill, McCormick was all in. McCormick's background in biology likely made her enthusiastic to be part of the wave of miracle drugs—aspirin, penicillin, the polio vaccine—which were changing the game of health and disease at the time.

While philanthropy was common among those with large fortunes, McCormick's choice to dedicate her funds to birth control was highly unusual. Even while public opinion was shifting, there were still laws that prohibited the sale and distribution of birth control at the federal level and in dozens of states. Being the only woman in her classes at MIT, McCormick was used to doing things that other people didn't understand or agree with; she didn't care what people said about her and channeled over $2 million to Pincus's lab, which would be more than $18 million in today's dollars. Sanger encouraged McCormick to spread out her wealth and provide smaller donations to a number of labs with potential, but McCormick wasn't interested in doing that. She wanted to see results.

In the end, the development of the birth control pill was funded almost in its entirety by McCormick. Yet she was more than simply the purse strings. Drawing on her own background in biology, she actively participated in the scientific development process, monitoring Pincus's progress and urging the research team on in their efforts. McCormick died in 1967, seven years after the FDA approved the birth control pill. While Sanger's name has gone down in history as the champion of the birth control movement, McCormick is the unsung heroine. Without her, who knows where the funding for the research would have come from, and how much longer it would have taken for the "magic pill" to become available to women.

The Pill Goes Viral

Once Pincus figured out how to create a pill from the synthetic progesterone (called progestin), he partnered with a Massachusetts-based gynecologist named Dr. John Rock to start testing the pill with patients in his private practice. (Remember that the FDA wouldn't adopt standards for clinical trials until later, so the way that drugs were tested with people was much more haphazard than drug testing protocols today.)

Rock was a devout Roman Catholic. He attended mass daily and hung a crucifix above his desk. He was fully aware of the Church's stance against birth control, but also deeply moved by the suffering he witnessed—both physical and emotional—when a woman became pregnant when she didn't want to be. He shifted to believe that women should be able to get birth control (well married women, he never went so far as to think birth control was for everyone).

In later years, Rock would go toe-to-toe with the Catholic Church on the subject. He wrote *The Time Has Come: A Catholic Doctor's Proposals to End the Battle over Birth Control* in 1963, arguing that a birth control pill that suppresses ovulation was not that different from avoiding sex during days when ovulation was most likely (a practice the Church did endorse). The book garnered him—and his message—national attention. So in 1968, when the Pope reiterated the ban against birth control in *Humanae Vitae (On Human Life)*, Rock became disillusioned with the Church and cut ties with his faith.

The initial small trial of the new birth control pill with Rock's gynecology patients was promising; the pill was working. So Rock and Pincus set their sights on conducting large-scale human trials with the continued financial backing of McCormick. With the Comstock laws still in effect, it was too challenging to try to hold the trials in Rock's home state of Massachusetts. Plus, Rock was concerned about following up with patients if they left their original location. Rock and Pincus also wanted to know if the pill would be acceptable in countries outside of the United States.

After considering several sites for the trials, they decided on Puerto Rico. In some ways, Puerto Rico was ahead of the game with regard to birth control: birth control was legal, and the territory already had a large network of birth control clinics distributing methods to women. On the other hand, the birth control infrastructure in Puerto Rico had a history of coercion and misuse. Puerto Rican women, for example, were often pressured to be sterilized after having two children. The pill presented an alternative for women who wanted to avoid both pregnancy and sterilization, but that meant many women felt like they really had no choice at all. If the only other option was sterilization, a reversible but highly experimental drug might seem compelling (though important to note that many women didn't even realize it was experimental either). Enrollment in the clinical trial reached capacity quickly. Rock and Pincus called their pill Enovid and began testing a high-dose version. After a year of testing, the first results of the trial came in: the pill was 100 percent effective at preventing pregnancy when taken correctly.

Unfortunately, that wasn't all that the first year of trials showed. Dr. Edris Rice-Wray, a faculty member at the Puerto Rico Medical School and medical director of the Puerto Rico Family Planning Association, was responsible for leading the trials. In addition to the high level of effectiveness, Rice-Wray also reported that the side effects of the pill were untenable. Seventeen percent of women in the study complained of severe side effects like nausea, headaches, stomach pain, and vomiting. Rock and Pincus dismissed this feedback, convinced that the women were overreacting and blinded by desire to share their miracle drug with the world.

Then the research team learned that the pill manufacturer, Searle, had accidentally been sending pills that were contaminated with small amounts of synthetic estrogen. This was a huge setback; the research team was unknowingly dispensing a different drug than the one they thought they were studying. Searle corrected the issue and sent the research team uncontaminated pills to continue the trials.

But the results were surprising. It turned out that the small amount of estrogen was actually reducing some of the pill's problematic side effects, like breakthrough bleeding. After further analysis, the research team realized that the hormones, estrogen and progesterone, worked together to prevent the body from releasing eggs from the ovaries and thickened the cervical mucus to make it more difficult for sperm to enter the uterus. A new version of the pill was born using the same combination of hormones found in pills today.

In retrospect, it is easy to see how problematic the Puerto Rico pill trials were. The rigorous standards for clinical trials did not exist back then, and it takes much more testing before a drug is even deemed acceptable for human trials. Further, much more follow-up is required when side effects or tragic outcomes are reported (like the three deaths that occurred during the trials). The women who participated in the trials deserved a lot better from the research team.

In 1957, the FDA approved the pill for the treatment of irregular periods and menstrual disorders and required a warning on the packaging that a "side effect" was that it stopped ovulation. Within two years, half a million American women had obtained a prescription for Enovid. Did all of them have irregular periods? Probably not. My grandmother got married in 1957 and was among the first wave of women who stormed the doctor's office for a prescription for her "irregular periods." The "off-label" use of Enovid for birth control was no secret.

In 1960, the FDA-approved Enovid for birth control, and by 1965 nearly one in four married American women under forty-five had used the pill. By 1967 there were thirteen million women using the pill worldwide, a number which grew to fifty million by the mid-1980s. Today, the United Nations estimates that there are 150 million people across the globe using the pill.

Controversy Ensues

The pill was approved right in the middle of the sexual revolution. A generation of baby boomers was coming of age and questioning the values and norms of their parents' generation. They marched against war, advocated for civil rights, and challenged the double standard that single men could have sex but single women should not. For social conservatives, their worst nightmare had come true. In their view, the pill was a free pass that encouraged infidelity among married women and promiscuity among single women.

That wasn't the only controversy surrounding the pill. Rock got the FDA to approve a high-dose version of the pill, despite the side effects reported by women in the trial. (In his view, preventing pregnancy was the most important outcome, and the high dose ensured that.) Before the pill manufacturer, Searle, could produce a lower-dose version of the pill, it had to prove to the FDA that the pill would still be effective with fewer hormones. Searle conducted additional trials that showed the pill worked very well at lower doses, and women experienced fewer side effects. Producing lower-dose pills also helped Searle increase their profits, which prompted several other major pharmaceutical companies to enter the market and start developing their own version of the pill.

Concerned about the reported side effects, Barbara Seaman, a writer and patient advocate, published her book *The Doctors' Case against the Pill*. She argued that women didn't have enough information about the pill and its side effects to make informed decisions about using it. Seaman's book prompted Wisconsin Senator Gaylord Nelson to hold hearings about the pill's safety in 1970. As a result of the hearings, the FDA required the pill packaging to contain information about possible risks and side effects.

Today, the combination of estrogen and progestin first used in Enovid is still used in a number of birth control methods: the pill, patch, and ring. The dosing of these methods is lower and side effects are more mild (though certainly not nonexistent). Researchers have also since proven that a birth control pill containing only progestin (no estrogen) is also effective for pregnancy prevention. There are many more progestin-only methods available, including progestin-only pills, a shot, hormonal IUDs, and an implant that goes in the arm. Estrogen helps to regulate periods, but removing estrogen reduces the risk of blood clots, a rare but serious side effect. (We'll look more closely at the menu of birth control methods later on.)

Making Birth Control Available—and Affordable—for Everyone

When Enovid came onto the market, Searle sold it at a premium. At the time, the annual cost of Enovid was the equivalent of about $1,000 in today's dollars, making it far too expensive for many people who wanted it. To fill this gap, the federal government stepped in to provide subsidized birth control, beginning in 1964 through the Economic Opportunity Act, a cornerstone of President Johnson's anti-poverty agenda.

Six years later, President Nixon signed Title X of the Public Health Service Act into law, greatly expanding the federal effort to make birth control available and affordable for all. The Title X family planning program provides millions of dollars to reproductive health clinics across the country. With that funding, clinics provide birth control as well as STI testing and treatment, counseling and education on reproductive health topics, and other preventive health services like breast and cervical cancer screening. People with lower incomes pay less, and sometimes nothing at all.

In 2022, reproductive health care providers used federal funding allocated by the Title X program to serve 2.6 million people—mostly women and people who are young, racially diverse, low-income, and un- or underinsured. Those reproductive health care services were delivered through a network of about 4,000 clinics across the country.

The Title X legislation was popular among both Democrats and Republicans when it passed in 1970. But since then, the program has been caught in the crossfire of the polarized American government. Between 1970 and 2008, there were 293 federal bills proposed to alter the Title X program. Attempts to restrict the program outnumbered attempts to strengthen it. Such ping-ponging makes it harder for reproductive health providers to do their jobs, and, more importantly, makes it more difficult for people to get the health care services they need.

The program got $285 million in funding from the US government in 2023. That's the same amount of money it has received annually since 2005. Can you imagine if you had the same salary for twenty years? Now imagine you are trying to use your salary to provide health care services to millions of people across the country. When adjusting for inflation, the program's budget has been nearly cut in half over the past twenty years.

Today, federal funding for birth control is dedicated to ensuring that people who want and need birth control can get it—services are provided regardless of someone's insurance status or ability to pay, and the program requires that all services be given voluntarily and free of coercion. Centering the dignity and humanity of people is core to the Title X program. But unfortunately, that hasn't always been the case. There's a long and not-too-distant history of federal funds being used inappropriately to coerce people to use birth control, or even to take away their ability to have children altogether.

Remember

- **First approved in 1960, the pill was born out of a partnership** between Margaret Sanger, who had the vision; Katharine McCormick, who provided the financial backing; and Drs. Gregory Pincus and Min-Chueh Chang, the research scientists.
- **The pill's release was controversial.** The clinical trials were conducted before there were ethical standards. The side effects of the original higher-dose pill were unacceptable. Lowering the dose resulted in fewer side effects and similarly high pregnancy prevention.
- **Even to this day, the pill remains hugely popular,** both in the United States and worldwide.

6

Shocking and Shameful

How Birth Control Has Been Used for Evil

It was a summer day in Montgomery, Alabama, in 1973. Two young women, Mary Alice, age twelve, and Minnie Lee Relf, age fourteen, were escorted by a nurse from their home to a hospital. The nurse was a caseworker assigned to the family through the federally funded Office of Economic Opportunity (OEO). Through the OEO, the Relf family, who were Black, had received housing support and other public assistance, as well as free birth control. The nurse had previously convinced the girls' parents, Minnie and Lonnie, that the girls should be on birth control because they had intellectual disabilities. The girls understood that they were heading to the hospital to get their next dose of the birth control shot.

The girls' mother, Minnie, accompanied her daughters. When presented with a consent form at the hospital, she placed an X on the signature line. Minnie was unable to read. She believed she was providing consent for her daughters to continue receiving the birth control shot. Minnie went home while her daughters stayed in the hospital.

Their sixteen-year-old sister, Katie, wasn't home when the nurse collected Mary Alice and Minnie Lee. Katie had previously been given an IUD without her or her parents' consent. When the nurse returned later to bring Katie to join her sisters at the hospital, Katie locked herself in her room and refused to go.

The next day, Lonnie and Minnie Relf attempted to visit their daughters at the hospital, only to be turned away. When the Relf sisters were finally returned home, their parents saw scars on their daughters' bodies. That was how they learned that the girls had been sterilized. They would never be able to have children. No one—not the parents, nor the girls themselves—knew what happened to them.

Involuntary Sterilization and the Eugenics Movement

The stories of Mary Alice and Minnie Lee Relf are two in a long line of people, primarily from historically marginalized communities, who have been sterilized without their awareness or consent.

The history of involuntary sterilizations in the United States is deeply intertwined with the history of the eugenics movement. The term eugenics—derived from the Greek for "good birth"—was coined by Francis Galton in 1883. Galton was disturbed by the fact that rich British families were having fewer children than poorer families. Inspired by his cousin Charles Darwin's work on natural selection, Thomas Malthus' concerns about population growth, and sociologist Herbert Spencer's detest for social welfare programs (having coined the phrase "survival of the fittest"), Galton argued that some people should simply not be able to have children, and that preventing "unfit" people from becoming parents would rid society of problems like crime, poverty, and unemployment. Eugenicist beliefs prompted discriminatory immigration policies in the early 1900s, as well as involuntary sterilization programs that arose around the same time.

The first involuntary sterilization law in the world was enacted in the state of Indiana in 1907. It required the sterilization of inmates of state institutions who were deemed "insane, idiots, imbeciles, feebleminded, convicted rapists, or habitual criminals." In 1921, the Indiana Supreme Court said the law violated the US Constitution and struck it down. But eugenics programs were thriving in the Midwestern states and in California, which performed about one in five of all involuntary sterilizations in the early 1920s.

In the early days, most people who were involuntarily sterilized were men. Vasectomy was a relatively safe and easy procedure, while cutting the fallopian tubes (known colloquially as "getting one's tubes tied") was not yet a mainstream operation, and hysterectomy (the surgical removal of the uterus) was even more complicated.

Learning from the failure of Indiana's law, when Virginia enacted a law in 1924, they mandated "sterilization of mental defectives" in order to promote the "health of the patient and the welfare of society." The statute argued that sterilizing institutionalized people would prevent them from passing down genes that caused intellectual disabilities, among other problems. This argument was not based in science at the time and has since been debunked.

Carrie Buck was just seventeen years old when she became embroiled in a lawsuit to test the constitutionality of the Virginia law. In 1924, Buck was sent to live at the Virginia State Colony for Epileptics and Feebleminded. Her foster family abandoned her there after she was raped by their nephew and became pregnant. After delivering her baby, Buck faced mandatory sterilization because she was diagnosed with "feeblemindedness." The diagnosis was likely a sham; the physician who diagnosed her probably scorned her out-of-wedlock pregnancy. It was extremely common for poor women to be labeled "feebleminded" as punishment. That label set them on the track for forced sterilization.

Virginia state officials wanted to know if the Virginia law would stand or be struck down like the Indiana law, so they convinced a lawyer to represent Buck and appeal her mandated sterilization. (Hardly a fair trial, the lawyer who agreed to represent Carrie was himself a fierce supporter of involuntary sterilization.) In 1927, in *Buck v. Bell*, the US Supreme Court upheld Virginia's law in a vote of 8–1. The decision gave states the right to forcibly sterilize people in the name of preventing the spread of "incompetence." Justice Oliver Wendell Holmes Jr. wrote: "It is better for all the world if, instead of waiting to execute degenerate offspring for crime or to let them starve for their imbecility, society can prevent those who are manifestly unfit from continuing their kind." Buck was sterilized later that year at the age of twenty-one.

With the Supreme Court's endorsement, involuntary sterilization programs grew. Thirty-three states had eugenics boards that oversaw the involuntary sterilization of hundreds, sometimes thousands, of people each year. People who had been historically marginalized were disproportionately targeted, including immigrants and Black and Latino people. Between 1920 and 1945, Latina women in California were 59 percent more likely to be forcibly sterilized than other women. In North Carolina, between 1964 and 1966, 65 percent of people forcibly sterilized were Black, despite the fact that they made up only 13 percent of the population.

The Virginia law was based on model legislation written by Harry Laughlin, a staunch advocate for eugenics. Laughlin wrote the model legislation to help states pass eugenics laws that would hold up in court. This model legislation was used by dozens of states, including

Indiana, which rewrote their prior law and instituted a new law that would stand until 1974. And when Hitler and the Nazi Party were writing their own laws, they turned to the very same model legislation—written by an American—for inspiration. It wasn't until the 1940s when the world learned about the atrocities of the Nazi regime and that there was a big enough outcry against eugenics to force states to get rid of their eugenics boards and stop involuntary sterilization programs for institutionalized people.

An estimated 60,000 people living in institutions were sterilized in the United States in the early part of the twentieth century. Nearly one in three of those took place in California, where 20,000 people in institutions were forcibly sterilized between 1909 and 1979, the most of any state. Virginia (8,000) and North Carolina (7,600) collectively accounted for another quarter of all involuntary sterilizations.

Having never been overturned, the decision in *Buck v. Bell*, which endorses the practice of involuntary sterilization, is still the law.

Out of Institutions and into Neighborhoods

But while forced sterilizations became less common in institutions over the 1940s, they didn't go away. Remember the Relf sisters? That was in 1973. And while not all of these sterilizations were done in quite the same egregious manner as that of Carrie Buck and the Relf sisters, it wasn't uncommon for people—mostly Black people and people of color—to be pressured, even coerced, to be sterilized. People who did not want to be sterilized were getting the procedure, and American tax dollars helped make that happen. How?

For some women in the 1950s and 1960s, getting sterilized could be quite hard. Up until 1969, medical professionals had a complicated formula for deciding which women were candidates for sterilization:

if a woman's age multiplied by her number of children was greater than or equal to 120 (to put that in perspective, a thirty-five-year-old was only a candidate for sterilization after having four children). And until 1970, leading medical organizations also recommended women consult with two doctors *and a psychiatrist* before sterilization. Several states had laws that required women seeking sterilization to have two children *and the written permission of their husbands*. But these recommendations had to change to catch up with the surging demand for voluntary sterilization. By 1973, sterilization had become the most common form of birth control for American women between thirty and forty-four.

Unfortunately, not all of those women chose to be sterilized. Because while it might have been hard for some (usually wealthy, white) women to be sterilized, poor women and women of color, especially, were being urged and even coerced into the procedure.

By the 1950s, the typical profile of someone who was involuntarily sterilized went from being an institutionalized man to a poor woman of color living in a rural area. Take, for example, Birthright, a nonprofit organization that provided sterilization services for young, poor, rural women, who were predominantly Black.[1] The organization pressured women to get sterilized by convincing them that they would be unlikely to be able to take care of future children. The women were basically guilted into getting sterilized, with existing and future children being used as pawns in Birthright's agenda: to prevent poor Black women from having children.

In 1948, Birthright fostered the sterilization of 150 women in North Carolina. They sterilized dozens of women each year through the 1970s. In the 1940s and 1950s, Birthright helped to set up state-sponsored "Human Betterment Leagues" (is that not a name that makes your skin crawl?) in North Carolina and Iowa, and a Human Betterment Federation that supported seven state leagues to fulfill their sterilization goals. The Iowa Human Betterment League sterilized an average of 150 poor, rural women per year from 1947 to 1951.

In 1970, the federal government expanded funding for clinics across the country to provide birth control, including sterilization. Some of that funding was used to coerce low-income people to be sterilized. Sterilization was proposed as a way to reduce poverty. The argument—poor people aren't fit to be parents—was a rebranding of the same one used by the eugenics movement a few decades earlier.

In Aiken County Hospital in South Carolina, for example, physicians refused to treat women who had three or more children unless they agreed to be sterilized. In 1973, thirty-four women who received public assistance delivered at the hospital. More than half of these women, eighteen of them, underwent sterilization; sixteen were Black.

In the mid-1970s, after receiving several complaints about coercion and abuse of Native Americans, Senator James Abourezk (D-SD) directed the federal General Accounting Office to investigate the Indian Health Service, which used federal funds to provide health services to Native American communities. The inquiry found fourteen women under twenty-one who had been sterilized, and seventeen women who reported they did not provide consent before they were sterilized.

Women would go to the doctor for one thing and find out after the fact that they had been sterilized without their knowledge. That was what happened to Fannie Lou Hamer, who went in for surgical removal of a uterine tumor, only to find out after the surgery that the doctor had also performed a hysterectomy. This practice was so common that it was known at the time as a "Mississippi appendectomy."

In Los Angeles, ten women filed a class action suit against the Los Angeles County-USC Medical Center hospital alleging they had been coerced into sterilization in the early 1970s. The ten women were low-income immigrants from Mexico, and all only spoke Spanish. All of the women reported that while they were at the hospital to deliver their babies, they were approached by hospital staff to be sterilized. Sometimes this happened after a difficult childbirth; other times it happened while the woman was in active labor. The women described being coerced into signing consent forms during labor, not knowing that the procedure was irreversible, and even, in some cases, that they were sterilized without their knowledge. One woman reported she learned she was sterilized at her postpartum visit, six weeks after delivery. Another woman learned she had been using an IUD unnecessarily for two years after being sterilized.

These were not isolated incidents. A doctor who did his residency at the hospital later wrote a report on sterilization abuse happening across the country and used his own experience at the county hospital as evidence. Between 1968 and 1970, he documented a 742 percent increase in elective hysterectomies, a 470 percent increase in elective tubal ligations, and a 151 percent increase in post-delivery tubal ligations. He observed doctors "selling" sterilizations, urging patients into accepting them, even reasoning with patients that they should get the sterilization because *the doctors needed the extra surgical practice*.

The lawyer for the women named in the suit ultimately obtained statements from 140 Mexican women who said they were sterilized without their consent. The women ended up losing the case in 1978. But they did succeed in getting bilingual consent forms in California.

As these cases started to come to light and the public started paying more attention, the government felt the pressure to act. In 1974, the Southern Poverty Law Center filed a lawsuit on behalf of Mary Alice and Minnie Lee Relf. The court proceedings unearthed hundreds of stories like that of the Relf sisters. An estimated 100,000–150,000 poor women were sterilized through the federally funded family planning program, and while the exact number of those performed involuntarily is unknown, even one is too many. The federal district court ruled on behalf of the Relf sisters. Judge Gerhard Gesell wrote, "An indefinite number of poor people have been improperly coerced into accepting a sterilization operation under the threat that variously supported welfare benefits would be withdrawn unless they submitted." He went on to say, "The dividing line between family planning and eugenics is murky."

In 1974, the federal government instituted new policies that applied to sterilizations paid for with public funding: a seventy-two-hour waiting period between the time when consent was obtained and the surgery (in other words, no more sterilizations after getting "consent" from a woman in labor); a near ban on sterilization for any woman under the age of twenty-one; and the requirement to have a signed consent form that clearly explained public assistance benefits would not be impacted by their decision to (or not to) obtain sterilization. But it would take another several years for these policies to be fully enforced.

Not out of the Woods Yet

The dark history of state-sponsored sterilization abuse is not just the United States' burden to bear. These policies have tended to target the most vulnerable people—the poorest, most under-resourced, most marginalized. Take China, for example. Because of China's one-child policy, an estimated 222 million women were sterilized. Wealthy families could afford to pay a fine to have more children, but poor families could not.

In the early 1970s, Czechoslovakia provided social benefits to poor Romani women if they agreed to be sterilized. In 1975, Prime Minister Indira Gandhi's government mandated that men with at least two children be sterilized. In the following two years (1975–7), an estimated ten million people in India were sterilized during what is known as "The Emergency" (the emergency being rapid population growth). In the 1990s, under President Alberto Fujimori, Peru coerced and forced 350,000 poor and indigenous women and 25,000 men into sterilization. In 2007, the United Nations raised the alarm on Uzbekistan for coercing women with two or more children into sterilization.

Unfortunately, sterilization abuse is not yet in our rearview mirror either. In the California prison system, 150 women were sterilized while they were inmates between 2006 and 2010, in violation of prison rules. Many of the women said they were coerced by prison staff. Even more recently, in 2020, dozens of recently immigrated women received hysterectomies without their consent while being detained at an Immigration and Customs Enforcement facility in Georgia.

Even today, transgender people face pressure to be sterilized in order to live the lives they want. Eight states and two US territories require that transgender people provide proof of sex reassignment surgery in order to update the gender reported on their drivers' licenses. Twelve states require proof of sex reassignment surgery in order to update one's gender on a birth certificate. In effect, these policies suggest that the only way to be a certain gender is to undergo sex reassignment surgery, which is desired by some transgender people but not all. Someone born female who undergoes sex reassignment surgery has to give up the potential for biological children, if they desire it. Some transgender people have to make an impossible choice between future family building and the ability to be recognized for who they are.

In light of the history of forced sterilizations in the United States, there are several protections in place today that make it harder to coerce someone into a sterilization that would be paid for with public funding. A standard consent form is used, and that consent form attests that the person seeking sterilization is over twenty-one years of age, mentally competent, and voluntarily consents to the procedure. The consent form must be signed at least thirty, but not more than 180 days prior to the sterilization; in the case of an emergency (e.g., a premature delivery) before the thirty-day time period, at least seventy-two hours must have passed since the consent form was signed.

Paradoxically, these policies that were created to protect people can also sometimes be a frustrating and devastating barrier for women who *want* to be sterilized. If they have private insurance or are paying out of pocket, none of these policies apply. A person can get sterilized tomorrow if desired. But if the sterilization is being paid for with publicly funded insurance, the sterilization may be denied because of an administrative snafu. Women have been denied sterilization and have become pregnant again, expressly against their wishes. Still, these policies designed to protect against coerced sterilization are absolutely necessary. Our history shows that we need these protections in place.

Remember

- **Proponents of the eugenics movement in the early 1900s believed that preventing "unfit" people from becoming parents** would rid society of problems like crime, poverty, and unemployment.
- **Eugenicists advocated successfully for the forced sterilization of tens of thousands of institutionalized people** primarily from marginalized communities, including people with disabilities, people of color, and low-income people.
- **Forced sterilization didn't stop when institutions ceased the practice after the Second World War.** Government funding was used to pressure and coerce people to be sterilized, and sometimes it was done without the person's knowledge and consent.

7

More Methods, More Problems

The Misuse of Long-Term, Highly Effective Birth Control

So once we had federal standards in place for sterilization, we stopped forcing people to use birth control, right? Sadly, no. As new methods came onto the market, similar patterns of misuse surfaced.

The Birth Control Shot and a History of Medical Mistreatment

Do you remember the Relf sisters, Mary Alice and Minnie Lee? In 1973, before they were taken away to undergo sterilization without their knowledge, they were already receiving Depo-Provera, the birth control shot. The problem with that: Depo-Provera wasn't approved for birth control until 1992, almost twenty years later.

Now, as you might know, it's not unheard of for medicines to be used for their "off-label" use. You might remember that Enovid had women rushing to get it for their "irregular periods" before it was later approved for pregnancy prevention. But, the story with Depo-Provera wasn't quite that simple.

In 1967, the FDA actually denied approval of Depo-Provera because of concerns about the drug's safety. In 1969, the drug was approved by the FDA—but only for noncontraceptive reasons, including the prevention of endometrial cancer. Despite that fact, 14,000 women at the Grady Clinic in Atlanta, Georgia, were given Depo-Provera for birth control between 1967 and 1987. Half of those women were low-income Black women. Many women who received the birth control shot during the experiment didn't realize that the drug wasn't yet approved and didn't understand the side effects that they might experience.

In 1992, when the FDA finally did collect enough data about safety and efficacy to approve Depo-Provera for birth control, that decision was opposed by prominent health organizations representing women of color: the National Women's Health Network, the Native American Women's Health Education Resource Center, the National Latina Health Organization, and the National Black Women's Health Project. These organizations opposed the approval of Depo-Provera not only because it had been given to women before the safety concerns were resolved but also because women of color had been disproportionately urged to use the shot for decades.

The testing of the birth control shot on low-income women of color was just one of many examples of egregious and inexcusable medical practice in the field of reproductive health. Reproductive health's unethical roots can be traced back to the origins of modern gynecology. Today, gynecology is birth control's "home" in the medical field. When you want to get birth control, if you see a doctor, you are probably going to a gynecologist. (You could also go to a midwife or an advanced practice nurse, but that is a bit beside the point I'm trying to make here.) The origins of gynecology are fraught with reproductive abuse, starting with the very founder, the man known today as the father of modern gynecology.

Born in 1813, James Marion Sims was a doctor who didn't have much interest in treating women until he one day encountered one who had fallen off a horse and was suffering from pelvic and back pain. Sims could see that the trauma of the fall had resulted in the tearing of a hole between the bladder and wall of the vagina (called a "fistula"). Today, obstetric fistula is treatable with surgery. But in Sims's time, there was no treatment. His first encounter with fistulas set him on a mission to develop a way to surgically repair them. In 1845, he began experimenting on three enslaved women, Anarcha, Betsey, and Lucy.

Enslaved women had basically no control over whether or not to have children. This became even more true for enslaved women in the United States after 1808, at which time the country banned the international slave trade, while the domestic slavery market exploded. Enslaved women were viewed as only as useful as their ability to produce more slaves for their owners to profit from. They were frequently and repeatedly raped by their owners, and when these women learned they were pregnant, it was not uncommon for them to attempt a miscarriage, preventing a future child from enduring slavery. For enslaved women, the choice of whether or not to use birth control was no choice at all.

Sims subjected Anarcha, Betsey, and Lucy to dozens of operations while refining his surgical technique. His treatment of the women was demeaning and egregious, requiring them to be naked and uncovered during the surgeries, which he invited other doctors to observe. The surgeries were agonizing, but Sims did not use anesthesia. He saw the enslaved women as undeserving of pain relief. This bias still exists. Black people are systematically undertreated for their pain compared to white people, a fact driven by untrue and harmful assumptions that people who are Black tolerate pain more easily.

It's quite possible that Anarcha, Betsey, and Lucy wanted to have their fistulas repaired. Fistulas can be painful, can lead to other issues like infections, and are associated with bad, stigmatizing odor. Women with fistulas are often ostracized. Yet, the women did not have the option to refuse the surgeries. The right to make decisions about their own bodies had been taken away from them.

After four years of experimenting, Sims did ultimately develop a surgical treatment for fistula. Even at the time, however, his methods were controversial. While Sims ultimately contributed to a treatment for a devastating illness that had no cure, the origins of modern gynecology are deeply rooted in pain, abuse, and exploitation. Like the use of Depo-Provera despite safety concerns at the time, Sims's work exploited Black people in the name of reproductive health.

The pattern of exploitation is perhaps most clearly illustrated by the infamous *U.S. Public Health Service (USPHS) Untreated Syphilis Study at Tuskegee*. In 1932, four hundred Black men with syphilis were enrolled in a study to better understand the progression of the disease. When penicillin was discovered in 1947, the men were denied life-saving treatment to complete the research. The Tuskegee syphilis study continued for thirty-five years *after* the discovery of penicillin, until 1972. By the end of the study, 128 men had died from syphilis or its complications, forty women were infected, and nineteen babies were born with congenital syphilis.

In 1876, Sims was named president of the American Medical Association, and in 1880, he became president of the American

Gynecological Society, which he helped found. Statues went up in his honor in New York City's Central Park, at the South Carolina statehouse, and outside of his medical school in Philadelphia. In more recent years, the statues in Philadelphia and Central Park were taken down. The Central Park statue was replaced with a plaque that acknowledged the contributions of Anarcha, Betsey, and Lucy.

The First Birth Control Implant: Norplant

In 1990, a new method came onto the market to much excitement and fanfare: Norplant. It consisted of six capsules inserted in the upper arm. (This method was a precursor to the current day implant that is just one matchstick-sized object.) Norplant released hormones into the body slowly over five years, providing a very high level of protection against pregnancy and a quick return to fertility after removal.

Many heralded Norplant as the first major breakthrough in birth control since the pill. There had been IUDs available before Norplant, but remember the story of the Dalkon Shield that caused women to have pelvic inflammatory disease and other disastrous health outcomes? That pretty much soured people on the idea of IUDs. Norplant presented a novel idea, and being a new long-term, highly effective method, it filled a previously empty void.

But then just two days after the FDA-approved Norplant, the *Philadelphia Inquirer* put out an editorial arguing that women receiving public assistance could be urged to use Norplant. "What if welfare mothers were offered an increased benefit for agreeing to use this new, safe, long-term contraceptive?" The idea of providing financial incentives for women receiving public assistance to use Norplant in the name of reducing poverty spread like wildfire, in the way that only truly bad ideas can.

When financial incentives make it impossible to make a decision truly willingly, they go from being potentially helpful (like providing rebates for eco-friendly appliances) to coercive and highly unethical—as was the case with Norplant.

There was a loud public backlash to the *Inquirer*'s editorial, leading them to issue a formal apology a few days later. But the idea was out there, and it took hold. This, despite the fact that Sheldon Segal and his team who developed Norplant came out vehemently in opposition to the idea, saying that the idea of Norplant was to *enhance* reproductive freedom, not restrict it.

"The line between incentive and coercion gets very fuzzy," said Segal. "The $500 bonus can be a heavy government hand on the scales of choice for the poor . . . When you single out a welfare mother, wave a $500 bill in front of her face and say the government is going to induce you not to have children, you've gotten into a risky area, ethically and morally."

In spite of this opposition, in the following years, legislators in thirteen states introduced bills that would provide financial incentives for women receiving public assistance to get Norplant. These coercive policies predominantly affected low-income, disproportionately Black women and women of color. In Texas, for example, legislators proposed a law to give women receiving public assistance $300 to get Norplant, and another $200 if they kept it for five years.

Going one step further, seven states introduced bills that required Norplant use, for example, for women who delivered babies with signs of substance use, terminated a pregnancy, or as a condition for receiving public assistance benefits. In South Carolina, a bill was proposed to require women with two or more children to start Norplant before being able to receive public assistance. In Mississippi and Ohio, lawmakers attempted to require women to get Norplant before being able to get benefits for their existing children.

Ultimately, none of these laws went into effect. But in the court system, there was a different story. Judges in several states—California, Florida, Illinois, Nebraska, and Texas—incorporated Norplant provision into sentencing agreements, and usually as a condition for reduced sentencing. Like monetary incentives, the choice of whether or not to accept birth control for reduced jail time is hardly a choice at all.

And at the same time, Norplant was heavily marketed to and even pushed on communities made up primarily of low-income women and especially low-income women of color. At one point, nearly half of all Norplant users were enrolled in public insurance, even though the overall proportion of people enrolled in public insurance was much lower. Across Planned Parenthood-affiliated clinics, while 12 percent of patients had public insurance overall, 90 percent of Norplant recipients had public insurance, meaning that people with public insurance were disproportionately more likely to be using Norplant.

Norplant was marketed especially strongly to young women of color. In 1993, students at the Paquin School in Baltimore became the first teenagers to be offered this method. The school's 300 students were all pregnant teens or new parents, and all but five of the students were Black. The Norplant program was designed so that students could easily get it while on campus. Some students (and parents) were relieved and grateful, but many others felt like the singling out of young Black women was problematic.

For some people, Norplant worked well. The high level of protection conferred over several years was exactly what people wanted, and for the first time, they could get. But for many other people, the side effects were untenable, plus it could be difficult to find a provider to remove Norplant. Between the proposed laws, the reduced sentencing agreements, and the heavy marketing of Norplant to low-income women, this method was forever tainted by its association with the idea that poor women, especially poor women of color, didn't have the right to make decisions impacting their own families.

A Balancing Act

Embroiled in controversy, Norplant got booted to the curb. By 2002, Norplant's distributor, Wyeth-Ayerst, stopped offering Norplant in the United States. To assume its place were some new (and also not so new) long-term birth control methods. The copper IUD, Paragard, had actually been around since 1988 but hadn't really taken off. The hormonal IUD, Mirena, was approved by the FDA in 2000. A new birth control implant, Implanon, was approved in 2006. By the mid-2000s, American women had options for long-term birth control in a way they had never had before.

But . . . they weren't using them. In 2002, just about 2 percent of American women were using one of the two IUDs available at the time. Around the same time in Europe, more than 10 percent of women were using IUDs. In Scandinavian countries like Sweden and Norway, it was closer to 25 percent of women. People wondered, why would IUDs be so much more popular in Europe than in the United States?

For a lot of reasons, it turned out. The problems with the Dalkon Shield were still fresh in people's minds, and people were understandably still cautious. Misinformation about side effects and risks, as well as who *could* get an IUD, was common both among patients and providers. Many providers hadn't been trained to place (or remove) IUDs and then the new implant. And then there was the cost. The upfront cost of the long-term methods could be hundreds of dollars, which was simply unaffordable for many people.

So researchers started to wonder whether eliminating barriers to the long-term methods would increase their uptake. One research team decided to test this hypothesis with the Contraceptive CHOICE Project. They enrolled almost 10,000 women in St. Louis, Missouri, about half of whom were Black and 40 percent were low-income. The team of researchers and medical providers partnered together to offer birth control at no cost to participants. Even the long-term methods would require no out-of-pocket expense. The first people to enroll in the CHOICE Project did so in 2007, *long* before the Affordable Care Act was a thing, so being able to get expensive birth control for free was a big deal. (It was made possible by a very wealthy anonymous donor who agreed to pay for the birth control methods directly.)

Besides getting free birth control, CHOICE Project participants also got counseling that covered the full range of methods. Counselors followed a standard script that stated the IUD and implant were the most effective methods.

The results of the study were astonishing. Whereas about 5 percent of women getting care at the participating clinic sites were using an IUD or implant before the study, "when the barriers of cost, knowledge, and access were removed, 75% of women in the study chose" one of these long-term methods. About 80 percent of women who initially chose a long-term method were still using it two years later.

The effect went beyond simply which method of birth control was selected, however. Through the three years of the study, people who chose a birth control method other than an IUD or implant were *twenty-two times* more likely to experience an unintended pregnancy compared to people who did. Because of this population-level protection against unintended pregnancy, participants in the study were half as likely to obtain an abortion compared to the regional and national rates, and they were also significantly less likely to get a repeat abortion. The number of teen pregnancies was 78 percent lower among young people in the study compared to the national average.

The data that came out of the study grabbed attention, and for good reason; it's not so often we can see such profound impacts with an intervention. I remember reading the newly published research from the CHOICE Project while in graduate school for a Master of Public Health. It was this study, in part, that attracted my interest in birth control and how important it is that people have *all* the options available to them, free of major barriers like cost. That idea motivated me to pursue a job working with reproductive health care organizations across the country.

In the following months, major health organizations like the World Health Organization, Centers for Disease Control and Prevention, American College of Obstetricians and Gynecologists, and the American Academy of Pediatrics put out guidance that encouraged counseling patients on the long-term, highly effective methods first. But in an effort to try to make sure that lack of familiarity with the methods didn't pose a barrier, some people started to promote the use of long-term methods—and especially for low-income women and women of color—too strongly.

Women expressed frustration about being targeted for long-acting methods, about being told that these long-acting methods were the best ones available, and about not being able to get IUDs or implants removed when they asked. "I told them that I wanted it out," said one IUD user participating in a focus group, "and they said that it's really expensive and that the IUD's the best option. I got some resistance there . . . I was a little emotional at the time and she [the provider] didn't even care, it seemed."

A study from as recent as 2023 found that 26 percent of women currently using a long-acting, highly effective method felt pressured to do so, and 11 percent who had ever used one of those methods felt like they had been pressured to keep it. Young mothers (under twenty-five years of age), low-income women, and Hispanic women were most likely to report this kind of pressure.

"All women should have the opportunity to make decisions about their own reproductive health and if and when they desire pregnancy," was how the original authors of the Contraceptive CHOICE Project put it. Pressure on women to use a long-term, highly effective method was counter to that goal. The balance between ensuring women could get effective birth control if they wanted it had swung too far in the direction of less, not more, freedom over their bodies.

Over time, American women have begun using the long-term, highly effective methods in far greater numbers than back in the early 2000s. Today, about 19 percent of women use the IUD, and 5 percent use the implant. There is much more widespread familiarity with these methods than there was two decades ago. Cost is less of a barrier, thanks to the Affordable Care Act, though the barrier hasn't been completely eliminated since many women still don't have health insurance.

In 2017, SisterSong and the National Women's Health Network convened advocates for reproductive health, rights, and justice to develop a Long-Acting Reversible Contraception Statement of Principles. They argued that long-term, highly effective birth control methods like the IUD and implant should be included as one "part of a well-balanced mix of options." The advocates went on to say, "People should be given complete information and be supported in making the best decision for their health and other unique circumstances."

The stories of forced sterilizations, abuses in the medical system, Norplant coercion, and over-promotion of long-acting, highly effective methods should forever remind us that people must be able to freely make decisions about whether or not to use birth control. There is a long, long history in the United States of powerful institutions making judgments about who should and should not be parents, and making it easier for some people and really, really, hard for other people to be able to have children and parent them. Generations of people have heard about or directly experienced these stories. Understandably, they have internalized anger and distrust for the system as well as fear and anxiety about being able to bring children into the world on their own terms. Will they be able to parent the way they choose?

Being able to build families if, when, and how we want to *should* be a fundamental right. Threats to birth control put this fundamental right at risk; birth control plays a role (not the only one, but certainly a big one) in exercising the right to build families. At the end of the day, birth control is a family building tool—whether the desire is to build a family of one or many.

Unfortunately, the right to create families hasn't been guaranteed for a long, *long* time. The misuse of birth control isn't the only way that the power to create families has been taken away from people. It's just the tip of the iceberg. For example, the fact that same-sex couples, people experiencing infertility, or people who want to parent on their own may pay upward of tens of thousands of dollars to be able to get pregnant because insurance doesn't cover fertility treatment.

Another fact: There is a long history of separating families— removing enslaved children from their parents, forcing Native American children into schools to unlearn their culture, and, more recently, separating immigrant children from their families at the border. Or the fact that about 700 American women die every year due to pregnancy or its complications, and they are disproportionately more likely to be Black, American Indian, or Alaska Native.

There isn't space in this book to go through the many, *many* ways that the right to have and keep families has been infringed upon.[1] This history might not be immediately about birth control, but it still impacts how people feel about birth control and decisions about family building.

Reproductive justice is "the human right to personal bodily autonomy, have children, not have children, and parent the children we have in safe and sustainable communities," according to SisterSong. Being able to get one's preferred birth control is one part of a world where reproductive justice is attained. The collective of Black women who framed the concept of reproductive justice in 1994 did so within the human rights framework. In doing so, they acknowledged the many difficulties that women—especially women of color and other marginalized people—face in being able to get birth control, other essential health care like sex education and prenatal care, as well as jobs that pay living wages and neighborhoods that are safe and free of violence.

And on that note, while there are many ways that women have had the right to create families taken from them, one that is particularly important for our discussion is that sometimes women get pregnant when they don't want to be. They simply can't get the birth control they want and need.

Remember

- **There is a long history of misuse of birth control.** Distrust for and anger against the medical system is one outcome of this history.
- **Reproductive justice is "the human right to personal bodily autonomy, have children, not have children, and parent the children we have in safe and sustainable communities."**

8

The Obstacle Course

It Can Be Really, Really Hard to Get Birth Control

Not too long ago, I was out to eat with two friends. Over pizza and wine, we swapped stories about our three young boys, all born within a few months of each other. My own son was coming up on his first birthday, and I felt like I was just starting to feel like myself again. We lamented the ratio of children's body size to laundry production (seriously, how do they do it?). We caught up on the neighborhood gossip. We shared summer plans. Soon, the conversation turned to birth control. I happily encouraged my friends to feel the implant in my left arm. (It probably won't surprise you that I do this a lot. It's arguably TMI, but I see it as taking advantage of a learning opportunity since in my experience most people haven't seen or felt one before. My husband gently reminds me that polite dinner parties are maybe not the place to brandish my birth control.)

After indulging me by tracing the outline of the implant in my arm, one friend said she was adamant she did not want to be pregnant again right then . . . and then sheepishly admitted that she wasn't using any birth control. Her doctor had said something that discouraged her from starting birth control before her six-week postpartum visit. Now, with a newborn at home, making another appointment on top of all the pediatrician visits just kept falling to the bottom of the to-do list. Oh boy, could we relate to that. I silently thanked my own midwife for placing a new implant while I was still in the hospital after delivery. Carving out time for the three of us to get together was tricky enough, and that was *after* all of the kids were asleep. Are there any doctors' offices open at 9 p.m. for appointments after putting kids to bed? Not around me, there aren't.

When people can't get the birth control that they want, they risk getting pregnant when they aren't ready for it. About four in ten pregnancies in the United States are unintended. The percentage of pregnancies that are unintended has gone down by 15 percent since 2010 (in part because more people are using very effective methods), but there are still a lot of people getting pregnant when that wasn't what they wanted. Admittedly, how people feel about pregnancy can be complicated. Some people are much more ambivalent ("it'd be okay if it happened, it'd be okay if it didn't") than others. Some people who get pregnant when they weren't trying for it will feel excited, grateful, and happy, so an unintended pregnancy might not be "bad." But other people will feel a range of other emotions: stress, fear, anxiety, regret.

About half of people who experience an unintended pregnancy are not using birth control, but the other half are. This says that however they might feel about an unintended pregnancy later, they were at least trying to prevent it to some extent. If someone doesn't want to be pregnant, they shouldn't be compelled to be—overtly or subtly. And if someone gets pregnant when they were trying to avoid it, well, it might feel like the world was pressuring them to be pregnant.

What keeps people from getting the birth control they want? Childcare, transportation, work—there are so many competing demands on our time that can make it hard to get birth control. Not to mention cost and insurance coverage, which makes birth control affordable or not.

Barriers to Jump Over, Hurdles to Jump Through

Many people who are postpartum—my two friends and I included—want birth control after delivering a baby. A screaming baby waking you up at 2 a.m. can be highly motivating for *not* having more children, but some insurance companies won't pay hospitals for an IUD or implant provided immediately after delivering a baby. The financial disincentive can be enough to dissuade hospitals from starting birth control right away, even when it's safe and convenient to do so.

Remember, too, that for people with public insurance like Medicaid, the waiting period and the consent form can be hurdles for people who want to get sterilized after delivering their baby (which can be a convenient time to do the surgery). There are other logistical problems that might come up, like not having an open operating room for the surgery. What does this mean for the women who wanted to be sterilized but couldn't? As many as 50 percent of women who do not receive a requested postpartum sterilization are pregnant again within a year.

When I was first prescribed birth control in high school, I didn't yet have my license. (I actually totaled my car on the way to take my driver's test, which scared the living daylights out of me and set me back a year before I was comfortable to try the test again. I did pass, even though my track record was clearly . . . not great.) I remember wondering how I would be able to get to the pharmacy each month to pick up my birth control. The closest drugstore was a ten-minute drive from my house. Oh, and the pharmacist on duty was the older brother of someone I knew from school. I lived in a small town, obviously.

I wasn't alone. Getting to the pharmacy to pick up birth control can be a real headache, and it can be a big problem if you don't get there. Missed pills or being late to swap your ring or patch can make them less effective. More than a third of women taking pills have missed taking the pill on time because they weren't able to pick up their supply on time. Some insurers have finally started to let people pick up several months of birth control at one time. Twenty-three states actually mandate insurance plans to cover extended supplies. And women who get a full year of their supply at one time are 30 percent less likely to have an unintended pregnancy than women who don't. Yet only 6 percent of women taking birth control pills in 2022 received a supply of at least six months or more.

In order to be able to pick up your birth control pills, you must have first gone to a doctor's office, had a visit, and gotten a prescription. At least that used to be the case, but all that is changing now. In 2024, for the first time ever, you could walk into a drugstore and get one type of birth control pill over the counter, without a doctor's prescription. That pill is called Opill, a progestin-only pill that can be 95 percent effective if used perfectly. Many countries have made pills available over the counter for years, but until 2024 it was only possible to get condoms and spermicides that way in the United States.

Only a handful of states, however, require insurance plans to cover over-the-counter birth control without a prescription. The suggested retail price for Opill is $20 for one month and $50 for a three-month supply. Without insurance coverage, that could be cost-prohibitive for some.

In fact, cost continues to prevent people from getting the birth control they want. One in four women with private insurance end up paying some of the costs associated with birth control out of pocket. While the Affordable Care Act required insurance plans to cover *at least one* of each of the FDA-approved birth control methods, just fifteen states passed laws that require insurance plans to cover *all* FDA-approved methods. So someone might be paying out of pocket if they wanted a certain brand of birth control not covered by their insurance (even though the insurance plan *should* cover it if the method has been recommended by a provider). They might also be paying out of pocket for a vasectomy that insurers aren't required to cover (the ACA only requires coverage of birth control methods for women). An out-of-network provider or pharmacy might also result in out-of-pocket expenses. Still, four in ten women don't know that most insurance plans are required to pay the full cost of birth control.

People without insurance can have a hard time affording birth control. One in six low-income women say that cost is the primary reason they are not using the birth control method they want to use. One in five uninsured women report having had to stop using a birth control method because they couldn't afford to pay the cost out of pocket.

Every year, health care clinics use funding from the Title X family planning program to provide essential health care services to millions of Americans, many of whom cannot afford to receive these services elsewhere. Unfortunately, there are also nineteen million women who need publicly funded birth control but live in a county without enough health care providers to meet the demand. Of those women, over one million live in a county without a single health care clinic that offers the full range of birth control methods.

Something else that is making it possible to get birth control without a visit to a doctor's office? Letting pharmacists prescribe birth control. Forty states have either implemented or were in the process of approving pharmacist-prescribed birth control as of March 2024. In those states, you can skip a visit to the doctor and walk into your local drugstore asking for birth control. Pharmacists with special training will make sure you're a good candidate for birth control, that you don't have any issues that would make it unsafe for you, and then outline the options they can give you right there.

On the flip side, in six states, pharmacists who are personally opposed to birth control can refuse to fill a prescription for birth control. (Fifteen states prohibit pharmacists from this practice.) Of the twenty-five largest health systems in the United States, ten are Catholic-sponsored facilities that can refuse to offer birth control and don't always provide referrals to other providers. In some rural areas, there aren't options for health care providers or pharmacists, so when someone refuses to provide it, birth control can be nearly impossible to get.

What are some other things that make it difficult to get birth control? The list is long. Nineteen states restrict people under eighteen from getting birth control without their parents' permission (unless, for example, they are married, have been pregnant already, or have already graduated from high school). Clinics that get funding from the Title X family planning program are required to provide birth control and other reproductive health services to young people without a parent's consent. (However, after a father in Texas claimed that those clinics were violating his right to raise his daughters the way he wanted, the courts stripped away the protection for confidential services in Texas in 2024. It remains to be seen what other states will follow suit.)

Not all insurance plans cover telemedicine, which can be used to counsel and sometimes prescribe birth control for patients. In more rural areas, low bandwidth means that even if insurance plans do cover telemedicine, it may be impossible to actually get a connection up and running.

Some people find it really hard to stop or change birth control—and it shouldn't be. Methods like the IUD and implant require a health care provider to insert or remove them. If people want them out, they shouldn't be told that it won't be covered by their insurance or that the provider isn't able to do that.

Some providers require patients to make multiple visits to the doctor's office to get birth control. This might include an initial visit to counsel about methods, and then a follow-up visit when an IUD or implant would be placed, if that's what the person wanted. When I first decided I wanted the birth control implant, I called my doctor requesting an appointment to get one. I was told that it was their policy to have a counseling visit with me first, and that if I still wanted a birth control implant, they would schedule me to come back for the placement. How annoying, I thought!

I had done my research and left my counseling visit exactly where I started it—wanting the implant. A couple of weeks later, I trekked back to the doctor's office to get it. Some people will undoubtedly change their minds during counseling (and that can be a great thing!), but even if that happens, it should still be possible to leave a visit with the birth control method you chose, no matter what it is.

One of my favorite parts of my job has been helping clinics around the country put systems in place to be able to do this very thing. That has included things like pre-making trays with all of the supplies staff need to do an insertion, which cuts down time for setup, stocking all of the types of birth control in the clinic, and giving staff easy reference tools they can use to check if it's safe for a patient to start birth control.

This has been satisfying work because extra, unnecessary visits compound the difficulties of getting to a clinic. It can be hard enough to take time off from work and get childcare for one visit, let alone for a second or a third one.

Beyond competing priorities like work and childcare, which make it challenging to get birth control, too many women experience pressure against (or for) birth control within their own homes. This looks like parents, other family members, or community members telling people to not use birth control. It also looks like people pressuring their partners to become pregnant when they don't want to be. This is a type of reproductive coercion that can also look like pressuring a partner to terminate or carry a pregnancy to term, using violence to incur a miscarriage, or destroying birth control—for example, flushing birth control pills down the toilet, poking holes in a condom, or forcefully removing an IUD—in an attempt to force someone into pregnancy.

In 2012, 10 percent of men and 8 percent of women had experienced some type of reproductive coercion. Men were more likely to report having a partner who tried to get pregnant when he wasn't ready for that. Women were more likely to report a partner had refused to use a condom. Black men and women were nearly twice as likely to have experienced reproductive coercion as white people. Young people are also more likely to report experiencing reproductive coercion.

Getting Rid of the Obstacles

Paying attention to the obstacles that we face when trying to get birth control is all the more important right now. In the aftermath of *Dobbs v. Jackson Women's Health Organization*, which overturned *Roe v. Wade*, states are passing laws that threaten our ability to get birth control, adding more obstacles that stand in the way of people getting birth control when they want it. Nearly all voters (96 percent) support the idea that women should be able to get birth control, and 78 percent of all voters think that birth control should be considered basic health care for women (this actually increases to 85 percent among women voters). Voters agree that we should be advocating for breaking down obstacles to birth control, not constructing more of them.

So what can we do in the face of these obstacles that prevent people from getting the birth control they want? One option is to get overwhelmed, frustrated, and demoralized—and that'd certainly be an understandable response. I feel that way sometimes. But the other option is to fight for our collective right to get the care we need.

What does that look like? For one, it looks like supporting strategies for making birth control affordable and easier to get—like insurance coverage for all methods, over-the-counter birth control, getting several months' supply at one time, and pharmacist-dispensed birth control. It looks like supporting a strong publicly funded network of reproductive health clinics to make sure that no one falls through the cracks, so long as there are people who are uninsured and underinsured. (And for that matter, it looks like supporting efforts to make sure everyone *does* have quality health insurance.)

To be good advocates for birth control, we need good information about birth control. Naturally, we all got excellent, in-depth coverage of birth control as part of a comprehensive sex education program in school. Oh wait, you didn't get that? No, I didn't either (and we should advocate for *that* to change, too). I remember some fear-inducing warnings about gonorrhea and chlamydia, the oh-so-classic "condom on a banana" demonstration . . . and that's about it. In 1995, over 80 percent of adolescents received formal education about birth control methods as part of a comprehensive sex education curriculum, but by 2011–13, this had fallen to about 60 percent.

Even if you did get great information about birth control back in the day, chances are there's been a lot that has changed since then. So there's no time like the present to learn the facts about birth control: what methods are out there, how to get and use them, how they work, and what side effects they have. And hey, maybe along the way, you'll realize there's actually something better out there for you.

> Remember
>
> - **There are *so many* obstacles that make it hard for people to get birth control:** Competing priorities (time, work, childcare), living in rural and under-resourced communities, cost, insurance coverage, and policies can pose barriers.
> - **There are some promising policies that are trying to remove these obstacles**, such as over-the-counter birth control, extended supplies, and pharmacist-dispensed birth control, but there is much more to do to make it easier for people to get the birth control they want.

9

Today's Specials Are

The Menu of Birth Control Options and the Many Factors That Might Influence Which One Will Work Best for You

There is no perfect method of birth control. How one person chooses to prevent pregnancy may work for them but not for others. The best strategy for preventing pregnancy is the one someone can stick to, using it accurately and consistently for as long as desired. Here are some aspects of birth control that someone (maybe you) might care about:

- Can it be easily hidden from partners, roommates, parents, or other people?
- Can it be obtained without a prescription?

- Can it be reversed or stopped immediately?
- Does it effectively prevent pregnancy?
- Does it treat other illnesses like PCOS or lower the risk of cancer?
- Does it have any negative side effects?
- Does it prevent STIs?

Each of us will answer these questions differently, based on our own needs and contexts. One person might be fortunate enough to not worry about needing to hide birth control from someone else; someone else may feel confident they are done having children and therefore want a permanent method. There are as many combinations of needs as there are people in the world. Fortunately, there are many methods of birth control to consider. Let me lay out some of the pros and cons of each method, drawing on my own experience as well as others who have shared their stories publicly.

Nothing to Remember, Easy to Hide—and Maximum Protection

When the Affordable Care Act's Contraceptive Coverage Mandate went into effect, I was in college and happily ditched the birth control ring that was costing me $50 per month. I wanted something long-term that I didn't have to think about, and finally, the ACA meant I didn't have to come up with a couple of hundred dollars to get it. It was free! I picked the birth control implant. I turned up at the clinic for my visit feeling excited. The nurse practitioner numbed a small area on my inner arm, slipped the little rod in, and bandaged me up. The whole thing took ten minutes.

The relief I felt was immediate. I didn't have to remember to get to the pharmacy every month. I didn't have to remember to store the ring in the fridge. I didn't have to remember to swap the ring out after three weeks. I didn't have to fret over that one time I took the ring out and forgot to put it back in for a few hours. And at over 99 percent effective, I could feel confident that I wasn't going to have an oopsie pregnancy that I feared would derail me from finishing my Master's program that I would be starting that fall.

For a lot of women, the most important thing in a birth control method is effectiveness—how good it is at protecting against pregnancy.[1] The most effective methods are "set it and forget it" methods. They are super effective precisely because they don't require someone to think about them, except every several months or years—one even lasts for more than a decade! These methods stand in contrast to a method like the pill, which has to be taken at the same time every day, or a condom that needs to be put on right before having sex (and in the heat of the moment, forgetting or skipping out on a condom is, ahem . . . plausible). The most effective methods are also the methods that are easiest to hide, for the same reason. What methods are we talking about here?

We've talked a lot about *sterilization* already. While there is a fraught history of misuse of sterilization procedures, they serve a really important purpose on the menu of birth control options. They are currently the only option for permanent birth control. There are three kinds of sterilization surgeries. A tubal ligation blocks the fallopian tubes, which is where the egg and sperm meet. A hysterectomy is the complete removal of the uterus and cervix. And a vasectomy blocks the vas deferens, the tubes that carry sperm. Vasectomy is safer and more effective than tubal ligation.

You might be interested in permanent birth control if you are absolutely sure you don't want any or any more children. That was the case for Emily, who shared her story about getting sterilized with the reproductive health organization, Bedsider. During her second pregnancy, she and her husband decided she didn't want to be pregnant again. She had gestational diabetes, was very uncomfortable during pregnancy, and knew that a third pregnancy wasn't something she wanted. Emily's OB tied her tubes during her cesarean section delivery.

Sterilization usually involves a few days of recovery; recovery tends to be shorter and easier for vasectomy. The procedures are over 99 percent effective: Fewer than 1 out of 100 people who have been sterilized will become pregnant per year.

The remaining birth control methods are all temporary, meaning they are reversible. One of those is an *IUD (or intrauterine device)*, which you've probably heard of, and since it is one of the most popular birth control options, you likely know someone who has one. IUDs are small, T-shaped devices that are inserted into the uterus by a physician, physician assistant (PA), nurse practitioner (NP), or midwife. In the United States, there are five IUDs available, four of which contain hormones and one of which does not. The nonhormonal one is made from copper (it is called Paragard). All IUDs are over 99 percent effective. Paragard lasts up to twelve years. The copper in it prevents pregnancy by creating an environment in the uterus that is incompatible for sperm to travel to the egg. Most women experience increased bleeding and cramping with their period initially, which generally improves over time.

The hormonal IUDs use synthetic progestin—a hormone that is very similar to the naturally occurring hormone, progesterone—to thicken the mucus in the cervix (which prevents sperm from entering the uterus), thin the lining of the uterus, and inhibit sperm movement so that the sperm doesn't reach an egg.

There are four kinds of IUDs that work similarly but vary in their size, dose, and the length of time they can last: Mirena (eight years),

Liletta (eight years), Kyleena (five years), and Skyla (three years). These methods might even last longer than that; research on how long these methods last is ongoing (case in point: Mirena was first approved for five years, but over time we've learned it actually provides a high level of protection against pregnancy for eight years). Regardless, you don't need to use the IUD for that full amount of time; you can get it removed at any time.

Having never had an IUD myself, I turned to my friends who have had them to give me the scoop. They've shared that sometimes the insertion can be painful with cramping lasting a few minutes or hours. But once that passes, people love how they never have to think about it. (While IUD insertion pain has long gone overlooked, fortunately the medical industry is starting to appreciate it more, and come up with better pain management solutions.) Because the IUD is inside the body, it can be easy to hide, though some people have told me that their partners report they can feel the string (more so in the early days, as the string softens over time). Many people have told me that they go months (sometimes even years!) without a period while using one of the hormonal IUDs.

By the way, if you hear that and the idea of not getting a period for months or years makes you nervous, you're not alone. Many people think that getting a period is necessary for something like "cleaning out the body." During a period, you shed the uterine lining, but birth control prevents the uterine lining from building up so it doesn't need to be shed. During pregnancy and while breastfeeding, you might also go months or years without a period. In short, if you are using contraceptive hormones it is perfectly healthy to not get a period.

Many people don't know that some IUDs also work as very effective emergency contraception. If you get a Paragard, Mirena, or Liletta IUD within 120 hours (five days) of unprotected sex, it prevents pregnancy from occurring immediately and can be used for birth control beyond that. After your IUD is removed, your fertility level returns to what it was before getting the IUD. Because everyone's baseline level of fertility is different, for some people that might mean you get pregnant right away, while for other people you might not.

You've heard me talk a lot about the *implant* (brand name Nexplanon) already. The implant is a tiny rod, slightly narrower than, and about the length of, a matchstick that a healthcare provider (physician, PA, NP, or midwife) inserts just below the surface of the skin on the inner side of the upper arm (near the triceps). Like IUDs, the implant is over 99 percent effective. It functions the same way as the hormone-based IUDs by releasing progestin. The implant is currently approved for up to three years, but ongoing trials show that effectiveness can last as much as five years. And like the IUD, fertility returns to "normal" (whatever that is for you) immediately after removal.

For me, I didn't love the idea of something in the uterus, but putting something in my arm felt totally comfortable. (I've heard people tell me the exact opposite, that the idea of something in their arm feels weirder than something inside them. Everyone is different!) You can feel the rod if you know where to look for it, but it's otherwise very easy to ignore and forget. For most of the time that I've used the implant, I haven't gotten a period, and that's pretty typical. Many women experience lighter or no periods; however, the most common complaint is irregular or breakthrough bleeding (spotting between periods, longer periods). When I do experience breakthrough bleeding, it is annoying, but it's also treatable with over-the-counter anti-inflammatories like ibuprofen or hormonal treatment (combined oral contraceptives or estrogen)—something you can talk to your provider about.

The *shot* (brand name Depo-Provera) is another longer-term, reversible method. When given every three months on schedule, it is also effective. But because it is possible to miss shots, the effectiveness drops to about 94 percent, meaning 6 out of 100 people get pregnant during a year of using the shot for birth control. The shot also releases progestin, working the same way as the implant and hormone-based IUDs.

You might be interested in the shot if the idea of remembering to take a daily pill is unappealing. That's why Alyssa, who also talked to Bedsider about her birth control, opted for the shot. While she doesn't love needles, she finds the trade-off between going to the clinic to get a shot once every three months compared to remembering a daily pill to be a no-brainer.

You may find a healthcare provider who is willing to train you to give yourself the shot at home (a practice that is more common internationally), but more likely you'll have to go to the clinic yourself every three months like Alyssa. The shot is very easy to hide, since there's nothing in a package and nothing in or on your body. If you do choose the shot, you might experience a delay in being able to get pregnant after discontinuing it. And you should be aware that the most common complaints are irregular bleeding, which can be treated, and changes in appetite or weight gain.

Stop at Any Time

While getting a very effective method that I didn't have to think about was the most important for me, that isn't what everyone wants. You might want a method that doesn't require you to go to the clinic to get it removed, as is the case of the IUD and implant. The methods that I'll lay out here require (for the most part) a prescription to get, but then they can be stopped at any time. This is ideal if you want complete control over being able to stop birth control, whether that's to stop feeling the side effects, to get pregnant (you return to baseline level of fertility after discontinuing any of these methods), or for another reason.

You are likely familiar with the *pill*. It remains the most popular method of reversible birth control. It's popular because it is so simple in concept. You just have to take a pill, the same way you might take an aspirin or a multivitamin. But unlike some other pills in your life, if you've ever taken the pill (or are taking it now), you know that in order for it to work right, the pill must be taken every day, as close to the same time as possible. The pill is 93 percent effective, meaning 7 out of 100 people get pregnant during a year of using it.

After one of my friends gave birth, she reached out to me to talk about birth control. She was breastfeeding at the time and was preparing for her postpartum follow-up visit, where she knew she wanted to talk about birth control with her provider. She asked me some questions about the long-term methods, like the IUD and implant, but ultimately decided to stick with the pill that she had been taking before she got pregnant. It had worked well for her in the past; she knew that they would be trying for a second kid in about a year, and she liked the idea of being able to stop the pill whenever they decided they were ready to start trying again.

Some pills are taken for twenty-one days followed by seven days of non-hormone pills (or no pills) during which time you experience "withdrawal bleeding." Withdrawal bleeding is not a period. You might be able to take the hormone-containing pills continuously (skipping the non-hormone week and starting a new pack on day twenty-two). This is called "continuous use" and can be used to avoid withdrawal bleeding altogether, which is safe and healthy to do. If you are interested in the "continuous use" approach, you should talk to your healthcare provider first.

Some pills contain only progestin, and others contain both progestin and estrogen that work together to prevent your body from releasing an egg (the estrogen also controls menstruation). The progestin pills work the same way as the IUD, implant, and shot; they are slightly less effective than combined hormonal pills.

The combined pills (with estrogen) have some added benefits: They can ease cramping, make periods lighter and more regular, prevent acne, and reduce the risk of iron-deficiency anemia, ovarian cysts, pelvic inflammatory disease, and uterine and ovarian cancer. The most common complaints are irregular bleeding, sore breasts, and nausea, though most women report these symptoms last for only a couple of months. You also shouldn't use the combined pill if you smoke and are over thirty-five or are at increased risk of blood clots.

Many people wonder about the hormones in birth control, while others have reservations about putting hormones into the body. Both progestin and estrogen have been thoroughly tested—for over sixty years!—and have been proven safe. The synthetically produced hormones in birth control are very similar to the ones that the body makes naturally, so similar in fact that the body recognizes them as naturally produced estrogen and progesterone. The progestin in birth control keeps the cervical mucus thick. If there is estrogen in the birth control, it regulates hormone production to prevent the spiking of the hormones around ovulation, preventing the body from releasing an egg.

Most pills require a prescription, however Opill (which is a progestin-only pill) does not and can be gotten over the counter.

The *patch* works the same way as the pill with both estrogen and progestin, and, therefore, has a similar profile of side effects and benefits. The patch is a beige-colored circular or square (depending on the brand) adhesive that you place on your butt, stomach, upper outer arm, or upper torso. The adhesive contains the hormones that are released through the skin. What I remember about my (brief) stint using the patch is that I was always worried that the patch would come off, especially on hot and humid days when I got sweaty during exercise or even just in the shower. It was the nervousness about it falling off that made me quickly switch to a pill where I had more confidence it would work correctly.

That said, for other people, the patch works just fine. If you use the patch, you have to put a new one on every week for three weeks. Then you have a patch-free week before starting the cycle again. (One version of the patch has a "continuous use" option where you can skip the off-week and avoid bleeding.) The patch is about 93 percent effective, though some brands of the patch are less effective in people with higher weights.

The *ring* also releases estrogen and progestin. The ring is flexible and a couple of inches in diameter. You squeeze the ring and insert it into the vagina, where it stays for three weeks and then comes out for a week. I used the ring for a while, and besides needing to remember to pick up the prescription and store it in the fridge, I didn't mind it. I forgot it was there most of the time, and it felt like a big improvement to not have set a daily reminder to take the pill. You can safely take it out for up to three hours in a twenty-four-hour period, which you might choose to do during sex.

The ring is about 93 percent effective. One brand of the ring (Annovera) is used for a year (you wash, dry, and store it in a case at room temperature during the "off" weeks). The other ring (brand name NuvaRing or generic EluRyng) is only good for one cycle, so you'll need a new ring each month. You may be able to skip bleeding on the ring by using the "continuous use" option.

The *diaphragm* is a silicone cup that you insert into your vagina to cover your cervix. It is a barrier that prevents sperm from entering into the uterus (there is also a similar option called a cervical cap that fits over the cervix, which is more effective if you haven't given birth before, though generally less available than the diaphragm). Remember how Margaret Sanger got her good friend Katharine

McCormick to surreptitiously transport illegal diaphragms from Europe into the United States? The diaphragms of today are new and improved versions of those very same. Look at how far we've come from those days!

Some people like the fact that a diaphragm doesn't have any hormones. That was what first drew Emma to the diaphragm. She also liked that she had complete control over the method (she decides when to put it in, when to take it out), and the fact that the diaphragm doesn't have any side effects. (The most common complaint is allergic reaction or irritation in the area; some people experience urinary tract infections.)

To use a diaphragm, you put spermicide in the cup and insert it before sex: you can put it in hours before you plan to have sex, and you can leave it in for up to twenty-four hours. It's generally not felt during sex, although it can be shifted out of place in certain positions. It's about 83 percent effective at preventing pregnancy. To get a diaphragm, you'll need to go to the healthcare provider to get a prescription, and depending on the kind you get, you may need to get fitted (one diaphragm, Caya, is "one size fits most" and therefore doesn't require a fitting).

Get It Today, Use It Today

I'm a planner. I'm the kind of person that loves to-do lists and especially loves adding things to the to-do list that I've already done so I can immediately cross them off the list and feel productive. I enjoy meal preparation and pre-scheduling workouts on my calendar. But I know that not everyone enjoys having a day that is scheduled down to the minute, and luckily, there are birth control methods that don't require much advance planning either. These are the methods that can be bought in a typical pharmacy or ordered online.

Condoms are cheap and easy to get, which is probably why they are so popular. Condoms are the only method (besides abstinence) that prevents STIs. They can be used in combination with other methods to both prevent STIs and provide extra protection against pregnancy. If you are the kind of person who gets embarrassed buying condoms in a store, the internet has done wonders in making it easy to buy condoms and have them show up right at your door. If you aren't the kind of person who gets embarrassed buying condoms, you get extra points for confidence!

When used on their own, external condoms are 87 percent effective at preventing pregnancy. There are also condoms that are designed to be used internally, which are about 79 percent effective (brand name FC2).

The *sponge* is a lesser-known barrier method. That might be because it has some tough branding. Does it sound appealing to stick something that is otherwise used to clean kitchen counters up inside your body? (For the record, that kind of sponge does *not* work to prevent pregnancy, so don't use that.) The actual birth control sponge is a small, round piece of foam that is inserted far back into the vagina before sex, so it blocks the cervix from sperm entering. It also contains spermicide.

You can insert it a few hours before having sex and keep it in for up to thirty hours. It shouldn't be felt while having sex. It's about 84 percent effective for people who have not given birth before, and the effectiveness drops to about 68–80 percent for people who have. (Childbirth can stretch the vagina and cervix, which makes it harder to fit the sponge tightly.)

Spermicides are chemicals that stop sperm from functioning once they enter the vagina. They come in several formats: creams, foams, gels, and suppositories. They all have their own directions, so be sure to read the packaging (e.g., some require a waiting period of a few minutes after they're applied). They're about 79 percent effective at preventing pregnancy. The biggest complaint is that they can cause irritation, and this can actually increase your risk of STI transmission, including HIV. There is a brand new vaginal gel on the market called Phexxi that doesn't increase the risk of STI transmission because it uses a different approach to stopping sperm from functioning, but in this case, a prescription is required. Other spermicides are available over the counter.

Emergency contraception stops a pregnancy before it starts. Pregnancy occurs when sperm meets an egg that has been released during ovulation. Emergency contraception prevents pregnancy by inhibiting this process. If the egg has already been fertilized by the sperm and implanted in the uterus, then emergency contraception won't work. But if that hasn't happened yet, emergency contraception can stop that process from progressing.

IUDs have been shown to be safe and effective when used for emergency contraception when placed within five days of unprotected sex, reducing your risk of getting pregnant by 99 percent after placement (and the IUD can remain in place for up to its duration after that).

There are also three types of emergency contraception pills, including one that is available over the counter. The over-the-counter emergency contraception pill has brand names like Aftera, Fall Back, My Way, New Day, Next Choice, One Dose, Plan B, and Solo. It is most effective if taken within seventy-two hours of unprotected sex (the earlier, the better). In general, emergency contraception pills can reduce the risk of pregnancy by 80–90 percent. Anyone can get over-the-counter emergency contraception, regardless of age or gender (though it sometimes requires asking the pharmacist to open a locked cabinet).[2] You can also order pills online from AfterPill (stock up now before you need them since it takes a few days for them to arrive). The other two types of emergency contraception pills are prescription-only (Table 9.1).

Table 9.1 Characteristics of Birth Control Methods

	Period Change	Effective	Start on Own	Stop on Own	EC	Permanent	Private
Nothing to Remember, Easy to Forget							
Copper IUD	+	✓+			✓		✓
Hormonal IUD	–	✓+			✓		✓
Implant	–	✓+					✓
Injection/Shot (provider or self-administered)	–	✓		✓			✓
Sterilization—Tubal Ligation/Hysterectomy		✓+				✓	✓
Sterilization—Vasectomy		✓+				✓	✓
Stop at Any Time							
Diaphragm		✓		✓			
Patch	–	✓		✓			
Pill—Combined Hormonal Pill	–	✓		✓			
Pill—Progestin-Only	–	✓	Only Opill	✓			
Ring	–	✓		✓			

Get It Today, Use It Today

Method					
Condoms		✓	✓		
Emergency Contraception Pill		✓	✓	✓	
Opill (over the counter)	—	✓	✓		
Spermicide		✓	✓		
Sponge		✓	✓		
DIY Options					
Abstinence		✓	✓		
Fertility Awareness Methods		✓	✓		✓
Withdrawal		✓	✓		

Key:
Period change: + increase; − decrease
Effective: ✓ + highly effective (99 percent effective or higher); ✓ pretty effective (90–98 percent effective)
EC means it prevents pregnancy *after* unprotected sex as emergency contraception
Start on own means you can get it over the counter
Permanent means you can't stop using it
This material is not intended to be a substitute for professional medical advice, diagnosis or treatment. The content of this table is provided for reference and educational purposes only. Always seek the advice of your health care provider.

The DIY Options

Finally, there are methods that don't require anything other than awareness, commitment, discipline, and maybe a little self-restraint. These methods have been around for millennia—remember Onan from the Bible?—and will undoubtedly be around for millennia to come.

Technically, *abstinence* is birth control, and it's 100 percent effective for preventing pregnancy and STIs if it's used perfectly—meaning you actually don't have sex. There are some helpful strategies that can make abstinence more effective, like building a support system, setting clear boundaries with partners, and establishing a backup (like having condoms on hand) in case plans change.

Abstinence works for some people, but abstinence-only education does not work. It fails to get young people to delay sex or reduce risky sexual behaviors. A major study that combined data on nearly 16,000 young people in the United States showed that abstinence-only education did not impact sex frequency, number of partners, sexual initiation, or condom use. On the other hand, when young people get comprehensive sex ed, they tend to start having sex later, have fewer sex partners, have sex less often, and use condoms and other birth control more often.

Withdrawal (aka pulling out or "coitus interruptus") is about 80 percent effective. It's easy to mess up because withdrawal requires a lot of self-control. It's easy to pull out too late or accidentally forget. You can use withdrawal with other methods for extra protection against pregnancy.

Fertility awareness methods (FAM) involve tracking the menstrual cycle and avoiding sex or using a different method of birth control on the days of fertility. (This can be used in reverse to time sex in order to increase the odds of getting pregnant.) FAMs take advantage of the natural rhythms of the body which is why it is sometimes referred to as "natural family planning" (though I don't particularly like that term since it makes it sound like other methods are not "natural." As we've talked about already, the hormones in birth control mimic the same "natural" hormones in your body).

If your menstrual cycle is between twenty-six to thirty-two days, you might adopt the Standard Days Method, which means using other strategies (e.g., condoms or abstinence) to avoid pregnancy on days eight to nineteen around when ovulation occurs and pregnancy is most likely to occur. Another natural indicator is the quality of cervical secretions, which, if checked daily, you can use to monitor when the body is most fertile. Your body temperature also changes during ovulation, so you can chart your body temperature each morning to determine if ovulation is happening.

I've had people tell me that their favorite part of using FAMs was that it helped them get to know their bodies more closely. You might also like FAMs if you like the idea of something nonhormonal. To me, the level of tracking involved in FAMs would feel like a headache relative to the "set it and forget it" implant to which I have grown accustomed, but I did use FAMs when trying to get pregnant and appreciated being able to feel like I was controlling something that otherwise is left so much up to chance. (And as you know by now, "leaving things up to chance" isn't really my jam.)

Practically speaking, you will probably need to make some purchases to make FAM actually work. Effectiveness ranges (77 percent to 98 percent effective) but FAMs generally work best when multiple natural indicators are observed and tracked. There is one FDA-approved app called Natural Cycles where you record your temperature daily, and the app will tell you if today is a fertile day. There's a special thermometer, called a basal body thermometer, that's most accurate for this purpose. There are other tools, like CycleBeads or a fertility awareness chart, that can help you keep track of your cycle.

Another kind of FAM is the *lactational amenorrhea* method (LAM), which, as a reminder, is exclusive breastfeeding which prevents ovulation. As a reminder, that means you are nursing every four hours during the day and every six hours at night, and that you are giving breast milk only (no formula) and directly (no bottles). LAM is about 98 percent effective. It's only reliable for six months, at most. Once the baby is sleeping longer at night, your period returns, or you start giving bottles or solid food, it's no longer a good pregnancy prevention method.

Is birth control safe while breastfeeding?

Yes. Hormonal birth control methods that only contain progestin can be safely started immediately postpartum and are safe for the breastfeeding parent and baby. That includes hormonal IUDs, the implant, the shot and progestin-only pills. Some hospitals will place the IUD or implant while you are there for the hospital delivery. Nonhormonal methods like the copper IUD, condoms, and FAM are also safe to start immediately (but avoid using a diaphragm or cervical cap until the first postpartum check-up). Methods that contain estrogen like the patch, ring, and combined pills should be delayed until four to six weeks after giving birth.

What if I Don't Want to Use Birth Control?

There are lots of reasons why people choose not to use birth control. About 40 percent of people not using birth control say they simply don't want to. Another 20 percent or so say they wouldn't mind if they got pregnant. The point is not to convince everyone to use birth control. It's that everyone who *wants* birth control should be able to get it.

Some people who aren't using birth control might actually want to be. The same study that showed that 40 percent of people simply didn't want to use birth control also showed that the other common reasons for not using it were:

- Being worried about or disliking the side effects (32 percent)
- Not being able to find a method they were satisfied with (11 percent)
- Not knowing which method to use (9 percent)
- Not able to afford it (4 percent)

If you want birth control, you should be able to get it. And that means being able to get a method that works for you. Anyone who doesn't want to use birth control should feel free to do that too.

Talk to a Health Care Provider

There are a lot of options for birth control. Some methods last for years, some for hours. Some have side effects, some don't. Most are free with the Affordable Care Act. Some require a prescription or a healthcare provider's help with placement. Some are easy to hide. None of them is perfect.

The goal of laying out the methods like this is to get some wheels turning. Hopefully, the next time you are at your provider's office or pharmacy, you have some more information to inform your decision. Or the next time you are talking about birth control with your friends or family, you are better equipped to share accurate information.

But this book does not replace medical advice. There are some conditions that preclude people from using certain birth control methods, and some methods carry a small risk of serious side effects. It's really important to talk to a healthcare provider about the priorities you have for birth control so they can help you find something that is safe and healthy for you.

It's common to try multiple methods before finding one or more methods that work for you. If you've tried something in the past and are feeling discouraged, know that there are a lot of other methods out there. A healthcare provider can help you navigate what hasn't worked for you in the past and find something that might work better for you now.

If you want to learn more about birth control methods, or compare methods that you think might work for you, here are a couple of my favorite resources:

- Bedsider: https://www.bedsider.org/birth-control
- Planned Parenthood: https://www.plannedparenthood.org/learn/birth-control
- The University of California, San Francisco, "My Birth Control" https://use.mybirthcontrol.org/

Remember

- **There is no "best" method of birth control.** Everyone has their own priorities and preferences. The best method is the one that will be used correctly and consistently for as long as desired. Every birth control method has pros and cons.
- **Sterilization, IUDs, implants, and the shot** are easy to forget, easy to hide, and offer maximum protection against pregnancy.
- **The pill, patch, ring, and diaphragm** usually require a prescription and can be stopped at any time. (Opill is a progestin-only pill that is available over the counter.)
- **Condoms, sponges, spermicides, and emergency contraception** pills can be purchased over the counter. (IUDs are also very effective emergency contraception but require a visit to the doctor's office.)
- **Abstinence, withdrawal, fertility awareness methods, and LAM** require some commitment and discipline (and maybe a few props).
- **Progestin-only and nonhormonal birth control methods are safe to use immediately after starting to breastfeed.**

10

Not Just for Pregnancy Prevention

How Birth Control Helps with Period Pain, Acne, Cancer, and More

When I got my very first prescription for birth control, it had nothing to do with sex. It had to do with zits. I was a teenager. I had them. And having them felt like the end of the world. When my doctor told me that birth control would help clear up my skin *and* make my period cramps less painful, I think I jumped for joy. Those cramps had me curled up in a ball clutching my abdomen and scrunching my face up in pain. Better skin and less pain? Sign me up!

While most people use birth control because it helps prevent pregnancy, four in ten people use birth control for the many things it can do that *aren't* related to pregnancy—known as "noncontraceptive benefits." One in six people use birth control *exclusively* for these noncontraceptive benefits.

Noncontraceptive benefits are a big reason why birth control transcends characteristics like whether or not someone is having sex. About 1.5 million women take oral contraceptive pills solely for the other health benefits provided by birth control, and half of these women have never had sex (young people make up a good proportion of this group). The noncontraceptive benefits of birth control lead people to use it, whether or not they have sex that could result in pregnancy (e.g., being in a same-sex relationship or having a partner who couldn't become pregnant or cause pregnancy).

Noncontraceptive benefits are an important reason—sometimes *the* reason—people choose a birth control method. These benefits are one more reason why it's so important to make birth control easy to get and affordable for everyone. Birth control is medicine, treatment, pain management. No one should be denied these health benefits.

What Are the Benefits of Hormonal Birth Control?

Hormonal birth control is one of the most studied treatments. The pill has been around since 1960, which means we have over sixty years of research about the hormones in birth control. Hundreds of studies have looked at the side effects, both negative and positive, of hormonal birth control. Because of this extensive research, we understand how estrogen and progestin provide noncontraceptive benefits. Methods that contain both estrogen and progestin (called "combined hormonal contraception" or CHCs) like some pills, the patch, and the ring have different noncontraceptive benefits than methods that only contain progestin (like the IUD, implant, shot, and progestin-only pills).

So let's go into these benefits, starting with the three most well-documented benefits of hormonal methods: cancer prevention, management of gynecological conditions, and lighter and less painful periods. Because I have been fortunate not to have firsthand experience with many of these conditions, I've relied on others who have publicly shared how birth control has helped them.

Cancer Prevention

Large, extensive studies have consistently shown that CHCs—methods with both estrogen and progestin—protect against gynecologic cancers, including uterine cancer and ovarian cancer as well as colorectal cancer. This is important because these types of cancers are common. Approximately 4 percent of women will be diagnosed at some point in their lifetime with colorectal cancer; 3 percent will be diagnosed with uterine cancer, and 1 percent will be diagnosed with ovarian cancer. Colorectal, uterine, and ovarian cancer are among the most common types of cancer for women (in addition to breast, lung, cervical, and skin cancers).

In 1968, researchers recruited 23,000 women and proceeded to follow them for up to thirty-nine years as part of the Royal College of General Practitioners' Oral Contraception Study. What they found was that women who had ever used CHC pills were 15 percent less likely to die from cancer than people who had never used CHC pills. Drilling down deeper, they saw that it was a few types of cancer that drove this reduction in cancer risk. People who had ever used CHC pills had a 38 percent lower risk of death due to colorectal cancer and a 37 percent lower risk of death due to gynecological cancers. Within the category of gynecological cancers, CHC users had a 57 percent lower risk of death due to uterine cancer and a 47 percent lower risk of death due to ovarian cancer.

In the United States, the Nurses' Health Study followed 167,000 women from 1976 through 1988. Researchers found that women who used CHC pills were 66 percent less likely to have died from ovarian cancer and 19 percent less likely to have died from endometrial cancer. (The endometrium is the lining of the uterus; endometrial cancer is the most common type of uterine cancer.) The reduction in the risk of death due to ovarian cancer even continued after people discontinued the use of CHC pills.

Numerous studies have replicated these findings. The UK-based Oxford Family Planning Association Contraception Study followed 17,000 women between 1968 and 1974. Uterine and ovarian cancer was significantly lower among women who had used CHCs compared to women who had not. Worldwide, CHC methods prevent an estimated 30,000 cases of ovarian cancer every year. When researchers combined the results of several studies, they found that CHC users had about a 20 percent reduction in the risk of colorectal cancer compared to those who have never used CHCs. Using CHCs for longer doesn't necessarily increase protection, but more recent use might offer more protection.

In addition to the well-established evidence that CHC methods reduce the risk of uterine and ovarian cancer, there is also evidence that progestin-only methods (i.e. hormonal IUD, implant, injection, and some progestin-only pills) and the nonhormonal (copper) IUD also protect against gynecologic cancer. For example, in 2014, a study of all women in Finland using progestin IUDs found that women using IUDs had lower than expected rates of uterine and ovarian cancers.

Management of Gynecological Conditions

When Robin was fourteen years old, she started getting bad periods. The pain from her cramps would be so bad, sometimes she threw up. Her periods lasted upward of ten days. She would soak a tampon in hours. She knew something was wrong, but she had a hard time getting someone to listen to her. She saw multiple providers who suggested she was exaggerating her symptoms.

By the time she was in her mid-twenties, she started developing gastrointestinal problems, which at first she didn't think were connected to her periods. She was nauseous all the time. Eating made her sick to her stomach. She met with multiple providers who suggested possible illnesses, but none of the treatments worked.

Finally, Robin figured out the problem after typing into Google her dual symptoms of GI problems and painful, heavy periods. She learned she had endometriosis, a medical condition where the endometrium, the tissue that normally lines the uterus, grows outside of the uterus, such as on the ovaries, fallopian tubes, or outer surface of the uterus. This tissue leads to inflammation and turns into scar tissue.

Pain is the most common symptom of endometriosis. This includes really painful period cramps, pain in the lower back and pelvis, pain during or after sex, intestinal pain, and pain during bowel movements or when urinating. Robin had been experiencing pelvic pain, pain during sex, and vaginal spasms, all of which she realized were connected to her endometriosis diagnosis. Endometriosis can also cause bleeding and spotting between periods and digestive problems (like Robin experienced), especially during periods. Endometriosis is also a cause of infertility.

It's estimated that about one in ten women worldwide experience endometriosis. It is most common in women in their thirties and forties, but it can occur in anyone who is getting a period.

What finally helped Robin with her endometriosis? Birth control. In addition to cancer, one of the most well-documented impacts of hormonal birth control is on endometriosis. There is no known way to prevent endometriosis and no known cure. What we can do is manage symptoms, either with medicine or surgery in some cases. For people who are not trying to become pregnant, hormonal birth control is often used to treat symptoms of endometriosis. Progestin causes the endometrium to atrophy, which reduces blood loss and pain.

Women with endometriosis who take hormonal birth control experience less blood loss, less pelvic pain, less period pain, fewer cysts, and less intense other symptoms. That was what Robin experienced when she finally got the Mirena IUD. The insertion hurt, but after a week's worth of cramps, she felt better. And when she experienced bleeding while on the IUD, she noticed that it was significantly different than before. She barely had cramps. She didn't feel nauseous. She used way fewer tampons. Her GI problems and pain lessened dramatically, too. In her own words, "The Mirena IUD made my life livable."

In addition to treating symptoms of endometriosis, hormonal birth control can also reduce benign ovarian tumors and ovarian cysts. Both conditions can resolve on their own and sometimes do not cause symptoms. For other people, they can cause discomfort or pain.

A few years ago, Planned Parenthood asked birth control users to share what birth control means for them. One of those people, Michelle, shared her experience as someone who gets ovarian cysts. "Ovarian cysts are painful and impair fertility. Without regular access to birth control (which I get thanks to Planned Parenthood), I would continue to have these cysts." She went on to say, "There are a variety of medical reasons that people choose a hormonal contraceptive. Regardless, every woman should be able to choose for herself."

Lighter and Less Painful Periods

Painful periods are incredibly common. Between 40–90 percent of women experience painful periods, and 10–20 percent of women report severe period pain. Painful periods are more common among younger women, women who haven't had children, live with high stress, and/or have a family history of painful periods. Painful periods can make it harder to participate in daily activities like going to work and school.

Heavy period bleeding can also be a difficult symptom to manage. Periods that last more than seven days, that require changing a pad or tampon after two hours or less, or involve passing clots the size of a quarter or larger are heavy enough to meet the clinical definition of menorrhagia. (Think you might have heavy bleeding? You can use the CDC and National Hemophilia Foundation's nifty scoring chart to see.) Even without meeting the official definition of menorrhagia, many women experience periods that are heavy enough to make daily activities a challenge. Heavy periods affect about one in five American women, or about ten million women annually. It's one of the most common problems that women report to their providers.

Heavy bleeding can lead to anemia, a condition when the body lacks enough red blood cells to carry oxygen throughout the body. Someone with iron-deficiency anemia might experience headaches and exhaustion. That might not sound so bad, but if left untreated, anemia can cause a weakened immune system, heart and lung problems, and pregnancy complications. And all that can come about because of a heavy period! About 6 percent of young women (twelve to twenty-one years) have iron-deficiency anemia.

Because painful and heavy periods can negatively impact physical health, mental health, and quality of life, the World Health Organization has called for menstrual health to be recognized not simply as an issue of hygiene, but as an issue of *health and human rights*.

Hormonal birth control is a treatment for heavy, painful periods. Progestin reduces period flow and lessens period-related pain.

Methods with estrogen make bleeding more regular; many women experience light bleeding consistently during the "off" week. Progestin-only methods (IUD, implant, injection, and progestin-only pills) can eliminate bleeding altogether (which, as we've talked about already, is totally safe and healthy). Some people experience unscheduled or breakthrough bleeding with the progestin-only methods; however, this bleeding tends to be much less than bleeding without hormonal birth control.

Jessica was someone who experienced very painful periods. "I have been on birth control pills for the past nine years to treat extreme menstrual pain," she told Planned Parenthood. "Since the ACA, I haven't had to worry about copays for receiving my birth control every month. And this has made my life much easier. Birth control is not just used for preventing pregnancy; sometimes women need it to treat a variety of health problems."

Young people report some of the worst period symptoms—and therefore stand to benefit a lot from the noncontraceptive benefits of hormonal birth control. A Swedish study of 1,410 adolescent girls found that 37 percent reported heavy periods, as compared to about 11 percent of reproductive-age women (fifteen to fifty) overall. In another study, out of 1,051 Australian high school-age women, 93 percent reported menstrual pain and 71 percent experienced cramping. One in four high school seniors reported missing school because of period pain. Another study of adolescents and young adults under twenty-six found that 41 percent reported not being able to do things they normally do because of painful periods.

Because period-related symptoms are more common among young women, they are more likely to rely on birth control for the management of these symptoms than other women. And don't forget about acne. It tends to flare up during puberty because of hormonal changes in the body and tapers with age, but many women experience acne into their forties and fifties. CHCs can help clear up skin and prevent excessive hair growth because they are "anti-androgens" (androgens are sex hormones; testosterone is one of them). Eight in ten women who are fifteen to nineteen years of age and using the pill say they do so, in part, for their noncontraceptive benefits, and three in ten of these women report using the pill *exclusively* for noncontraceptive reasons.

"Without birth control, I'd never be able to get through college," Jesse told Planned Parenthood when asked how birth control impacted her life. "Also, it does more than prevent unwanted pregnancies. Without it, every month I would spend one entire week in severe pain. This not only regulates my period but helps me function in my everyday life."

Another time in one's life that hormonal birth control's noncontraceptive benefits may be helpful is during perimenopause. Once someone reaches menopause, they stop having a period (and have officially reached menopause if they haven't had a period in twelve months). Perimenopause starts before then—typically in a person's forties and fifties—and can last for years. During perimenopause, the periods might be all over the place: no period for a few months then—boom—it comes back. It can be hard for someone to know when to stop worrying about getting pregnant.

For Lori, that was the reason she decided to use birth control. "My OB-GYN has prescribed birth control pills for me, a woman nearly fifty-two years of age, as part of my treatment for perimenopausal symptoms," she told Planned Parenthood. "It is highly unlikely that I would become pregnant at my age, but it is still physically possible. I appreciate the fact that I have access to birth control for both reasons." Hormonal birth control can help someone prevent pregnancy while also regulating periods and reducing period pain and bleeding.

Other Benefits

The pain and bleeding management provided by birth control can be extended to manage other conditions, like gender dysphoria and period-related symptoms.

Gender Dysphoria

Transgender men may use hormonal birth control to avoid getting a period and prevent an unplanned pregnancy. Getting a period as a transgender man can cause feelings of gender dysphoria (which is stress or discomfort caused by the fact that the gender you identify with does not align with the sex you were born with). Hormonal birth control methods that are taken continuously and therefore eliminate bleeding can suppress those feelings. All forms of birth control can help prevent an unplanned pregnancy, which can also trigger gender dysphoria.

After a stressful pregnancy that ended with a miscarriage, Zachary, a transgender man, decided to use birth control. He shared his story with the National Women's Law Center to help them advocate for birth control. "Going through that was very difficult, as I had to deal with both gender dysphoria and the depression that comes from a miscarriage, especially when I couldn't tell anyone. Hormonal birth control helps me take control over my body and prevent pregnancy."

On the other hand, when there is breakthrough or unscheduled bleeding with those methods, it can worsen feelings of gender dysphoria. Taking "female" hormones like estrogen can also complicate feelings about birth control.

Given that there are a lot of factors that might influence a transgender person's need for and desire to take hormonal birth control—the same of which is true for cisgender people—sometimes it is necessary to try a few different types of birth control to find one that works best.

Period-related Symptoms

Some types of CHCs also reduce premenstrual dysphoric disorder (PMDD), which is a more serious form of premenstrual syndrome (PMS). People with PMDD experience typical PMS symptoms (like bloating, headaches, and breast tenderness) as well as extreme irritability, anxiety, mood changes, and depression. PMDD affects as many as one in ten people who get periods.

"When I was a high school student, even before I became sexually active, birth control pills helped me and many of my friends who suffered debilitating cramps and mood swings," Jessica told Planned Parenthood when asked about how birth control impacted her. "Today birth control helps me plan for a future I can afford, without unplanned pregnancies which, as an unemployed graduate student, would derail my academic and financial future."

What Are the Side Effects and Risks Associated with Hormonal Birth Control?

Many people don't experience negative side effects with hormonal birth control. But some people do. It's completely normal to be concerned about side effects of medications. One in three people not using birth control say it's because of side effects. So what exactly are these side effects, and how common are they?

Most Common Side Effects

The birth control implant has worked great for me. I love that I never have to think about it. It's always there, doing the work behind the scenes. But one thing I don't love: getting random bleeding. Because the birth control implant is used continuously (versus something like the pill where you might have a week off), bleeding is completely unscheduled, and it always catches me off guard. I have gone several months without any bleeding. Those months are great! Then there might be a month where there are a handful of times when bleeding catches me unprepared. Those months are . . . not so great.

Unscheduled or breakthrough bleeding is the most common side effect of progestin-only methods. The CDC recommends five to seven days of NSAIDs (such as ibuprofen) to treat unscheduled bleeding. Another treatment option is temporarily taking a CHC pill (which requires a prescription). When that pesky bleeding catches me off guard, I start a regimen of ibuprofen. It doesn't always work, but I'm grateful when it does. And most people I know who experience breakthrough bleeding don't know that this is a treatment option that they can talk to their health care provider about.

About 10 percent of people taking CHCs experience nausea, breast tenderness, and headaches—the most common side effects. Usually, those symptoms resolve on their own within a couple of months. When they don't resolve, one option is to try a different type of birth control with a different dose and even different versions of the hormones. Sometimes, the body tolerates one method better than another.

Rare but Serious Side Effects

One of the most significant negative side effects of CHCs is venous thromboembolism (VTE), when blood clots form in the veins. Untreated, blood clots can restrict blood flow and oxygen through the body, which can lead to organ or tissue damage. It's especially serious if a blood clot blocks blood from flowing to the lungs (a "pulmonary embolism"), which can result in death. While VTE is a serious concern, the overall risk of VTE is very, very small—with or without CHCs. Still, CHCs aren't recommended for people who have hypertension or who smoke and are over thirty-five, because these factors make people more susceptible to blood clots. Progestin-only methods don't increase the risk of VTE, so they are considered safer for people who have a higher risk of getting blood clots.

Where the Data Is Less Clear

Some studies have shown that using CHCs is associated with a higher risk of breast cancer. However, the quality of these studies has not been as strong with notable limitations, for example, focusing only on women with BRCA1 and BRCA2 genes who have an inherently higher risk of breast cancer, or failing to take into account behaviors like alcohol consumption and physical activity which also impact breast cancer risk. The overall risk of breast cancer is low, and the increased risk of CHCs translates to about one additional case of invasive breast cancer for every 7,690 women using hormonal contraception. Because CHCs protect against other types of cancer, someone's overall cancer risk may still be less if they use CHCs, even after accounting for a slight increase in the risk of breast cancer.

There is also mixed data about cervical cancer. Some studies show a slight increase in the risk of cervical cancer among people using CHCs for five or more years. But the quality of this data is also low. Importantly, few studies looking at cervical cancer risk have controlled for HPV ("human papillomavirus") infection status, which increases someone's risk of cervical cancer. The risk of cervical cancer seems to decline after stopping the use of CHCs.

(While we are on the subject of cervical cancer, I would be remiss if I didn't take this opportunity to plug the HPV vaccine. The HPV

Table 10.1 Summary of Noncontraceptive Benefits

Noncontraceptive Benefit	Methods with Estrogen and Progestin	Methods with Only Progestin (No Estrogen)				Nonhormonal Methods	
	CHC Pills, Patch, Ring	Hormonal IUD	Implant	Injection	Progestin-Only Pills	Condom	Copper IUD
Prevents cancers:							
Uterine (endometrial)	✓	✓	✓				✓
Ovarian	✓	✓	✓	✓	Some		
Colorectal	✓						
Cervical							✓
Treats gynecological conditions, pain, and heavy bleeding:							
Endometriosis	✓	✓	✓	✓			
Heavy and painful periods, anemia	✓	✓	✓	✓	✓		
Premenstrual dysphoric disorder	✓						
Protects against:							
Feelings of gender dysphoria	?	?	?	?	?		
Acne, excess hair	✓						
Sexually transmitted infections						✓	

vaccine [Gardasil 9] prevents nine types of HPV that cause 80–90 percent of cervical cancers. The good news is that the percentage of adolescents who have received the HPV vaccine is increasing. In 2022, more than half of both adolescent boys [57 percent] and girls [60 percent] had received the recommended two or three doses of the vaccine. There's still a lot of work to be done; Table 10.1.)

Condoms and STI Prevention

Hormonal birth control can do a lot of things, but one thing it can't do is prevent STIs. The only birth control method available that can do that is the condom. (Although researchers are working on other ways of preventing STIs, so that may soon be changing. I'll come back to this shortly.)

This matters a lot because STIs are extremely common. Over half of Americans will get an STI other than HIV in their lifetime. In 2018, the CDC estimated that about one in five people currently has an STI. That translates to approximately seventy million infections. About twenty-six million Americans get a new STI each year. Nearly half of those new infections occur in young people ages fifteen to twenty-four. Young people, people living in under-resourced communities including people of color, and people who identify as LGBTQIA+[1] disproportionately carry the burden of STIs. Societal level factors, including stigma surrounding STIs, poverty, oppression, and access to health care, influence whether and how people experience STI prevention, testing, and treatment.

These should sound like high numbers, because they are. And they are getting higher. Since 2000, the number of gonorrhea cases has increased 78 percent, and chlamydia cases have increased 133 percent. Syphilis cases are more than five times higher today than they were in 2000. One of the many negative consequences of the pandemic was that people were prevented from getting timely diagnosis and treatment of STIs.[2]

In the words of the director of the National Coalition of STD Directors, "The latest CDC data shows record high STI rates in America for the eighth straight year. This is not business as usual—it is a rapidly deteriorating public health crisis in a dangerous time."

Untreated, STIs can lead to major health problems. So early detection is important—and prevention is even better. Vaccines can protect against a few STIs (HPV, hepatitis) and there's a medication to prevent HIV (called PrEP), but for the most part, condoms are our best STI prevention strategy. And, we could be doing better when it comes to using condoms consistently. Six in ten people say they used a condom the first time they had sex. One in four women and one in three men ages fifteen to forty-nine report using a condom every time.[3] In 2019, just about half of high school students said they used a condom the last time they had sex. And 9 percent of high schoolers said they used condoms along with another form of birth control for pregnancy prevention.

Birth control confers a wide range of benefits: from pregnancy prevention to the treatment of medical conditions to cancer prevention. At an individual level, the benefits of birth control can change lives. Nearly everyone has a story about what birth control has meant for them personally. Maybe it meant they could finish school before starting a family. Maybe it meant they could resume daily activities after treating unbearable period pain. So what happens when you add up all the benefits that each of us experiences from using birth control and look at the sum of those benefits across communities? When you do that, you see that birth control doesn't just change lives; it changes societies.

Remember

- **Many people use birth control for reasons unrelated to preventing pregnancy.**

- **Hormonal birth control has many noncontraceptive benefits** including: reducing the risk of colorectal, uterine and ovarian cancer; managing symptoms of gynecological conditions; and making periods lighter and less painful.

- A lot of people do not experience ongoing side effects of birth control, but the **most common side effects are things like nausea, breast tenderness, headaches, and unscheduled bleeding.** There are also some rare but serious side effects of birth control.

- **Condoms are the only birth control method that prevents both pregnancy and STIs.** STIs are very common and in many cases, increasing. Early identification is good, but prevention is better.

11

Changing Lives, Changing Societies

How Birth Control Has Changed the World

At the turn of the century, as revelers donned their year 2000 glasses and everyone fretted about the impending Y2K bug, the Centers for Disease Control and Prevention, like many of us are inclined to do at the end of an era, reflected on the past and considered the future. Researchers and staff looked back over a hundred years of science, advancements, and stories to identify the ten greatest public health achievements of the twentieth century. It was a hard task, given just how momentous that century was for public health. Between 1900 and 1999, the average lifespan of an American increased by thirty years, from about forty-eight to seventy-six years of age. Over 80 percent of that improvement, twenty-five years, was attributable to public health policies, innovations, campaigns, and oversight.

What were the public health advancements that we can thank for the dramatic increase in life expectancy? The list, in no particular order, includes some heavy hitters (arguably, the *heaviest* hitters of them all): vaccines that eradicated smallpox, eliminated polio in the United States, and made common and deadly diseases like measles, rubella, tetanus, and diphtheria a thing of the past for most Americans. Also on the list: large declines in motor vehicle-related deaths due to safer vehicles and roads, and increased use of safety belts and motorcycle helmets.

The list continues with safer workplaces and fewer worksite-related injuries and deaths. Clean water and sanitation that dramatically reduced the spread of infectious diseases like typhoid and cholera. A large reduction (51 percent) in deaths from heart disease. Safer foods free from contamination and fortified to prevent diseases associated with nutritional deficiency.

Enormous reductions in infant mortality (90 percent) and maternal mortality (99 percent) have occurred since the turn of the century. Fluoridation in drinking water began in 1945 and resulted in over 40 percent reductions in tooth decay in children and tooth loss in adults. There is recognition of the myriad problems caused by tobacco use, along with successful tobacco cessation efforts.

And the tenth greatest public health achievements of the twentieth century in the United States? Well of course you knew when we started down this road what it was going to be, didn't you? Birth control. In the words of the CDC, "Access to family planning and contraceptive services has altered social and economic roles of women." Just how important has birth control been to society? Like the other advancements on the list, birth control might not be flashy. But quietly in the background, it has been contributing to a safer, healthier, more gender-equal world.

Birth Control Helps People Choose If and When to Have Children

So what exactly does the availability of birth control have to do with the social and economic roles of women? It might seem like a big leap to go from preventing pregnancy to advancing women's role in society, and certainly, the introduction of birth control was not the *only* contributor that moved us to the more gender-equal society we have today. But it played a big role, and the first thing that the introduction of birth control did was help women decide if and when to have children.

It may seem like a foregone conclusion that greater access to birth control would result in fewer pregnancies and births. Yet, in the world of science and data, nothing is ever considered a foregone conclusion, especially when we're trying to make conclusions about major societal changes. (In fact, when we *do* assume outcomes based on "common sense," we can get in trouble. Remember that before we examined the health impacts of smoking, cigarettes were thought to be healthy in the absence of any proof otherwise.)

In 1965, the Supreme Court struck down Connecticut's birth control ban, legalizing birth control for married people across the country. Before the *Griswold v. Connecticut* decision, some states had already legalized birth control, while others, like Connecticut, had not. So when the pill was approved in 1960, women living in states where birth control was legal had a much easier time getting it than women living in states where it was not. This situation presents a sort of natural experiment for evaluating the impact of birth control. In states with no ban on birth control, we would expect the Griswold ruling to have no impact; women continued to have access to birth control. In states with a ban on birth control, we'd expect the newfound access to birth control that came with the ruling to have a big effect.

When looking at the data in this way, what you see is that women living in states where birth control was legal had fewer children than women living in states where it was illegal. When the *Griswold v. Connecticut* decision legalized birth control everywhere, the women who had previously been denied birth control could now get it—started having fewer children too. All told, researchers estimate that as much as 40 percent of the decline in the number of children married couples had between 1955 and 1965 can be attributed to the pill.

Flash forward to the current day. Birth control has also contributed to the reduction in teen pregnancies over the past few decades. Raising kids can be challenging at any age, and teen parents in particular don't get a lot of support, which is part of the reason this measure is looked at so closely. The number of pregnant teens has gone down about 75 percent since it peaked in 1991. (But teen pregnancy is still more common in the United States than in countries like Canada, France, and Germany which provide better sex education and more social support for teens.) Part of this decline is because more young people are using birth control consistently and correctly, including some of the most effective methods like the IUD and implant. In 2002, less than 1 percent of young women (fifteen to nineteen years old) used the IUD or implant. By 2019, that had increased to nearly 20 percent. By some estimates, increased use of birth control among young people accounts for 86 percent of the decline in teen births.

More Options for Women

As women were able to take more control over their fertility, suddenly they had options they didn't have before. One option that became available? Higher education.

The launch of the pill helped more women go to college. We know this because of another natural experiment. After the pill was legalized, some states required women to be twenty-one to get it, while in other states women only needed to be eighteen. Over time, all states dropped the age to eighteen. But since states lowered the age at different times, researchers were able to compare how laws around age requirements impacted how much education women got. Even though the difference was just three years (between the ages of eighteen and twenty-one), this period is a critical time to decide whether to pursue higher education—so there were noticeable impacts.

College enrollment, it turns out, was 20 percent higher among women in their early twenties who had early legal access to birth control, compared to women who did not. Whereas before women might not have even considered college because they were or expected to soon be pregnant—or may have dropped out of college upon getting pregnant—now they could see a future that included early education, and they went for it. Women with early legal access to the pill attended an average of one more year of higher education before age thirty. This was just the beginning; since then more and more women have gone on to higher education. Since the mid-1960s, the gap between men and women having a college degree has shrunk steadily. And today, women are actually more likely to complete college than men (39 percent vs. 36 percent).

The pill also helped women who enrolled in college to stay in college. Women who had early legal access to the pill had a 35 percent lower dropout rate compared to women who did not.

Researchers estimate that about one third of the rise in women's enrollment in college from 1969 to 1980 can be attributed to access to the pill. My mother enrolled in college in the fall of 1976, right in the midst of this sea change. She was one of the first 129 women to be admitted as first-year students to the college. In her freshman class, men outnumbered women two to one. She would be the first to say that this was not an easy dynamic. Not all of the men in her class were happy to see women in their classes, taking the seats from the men who would otherwise have been there. It was lonely and isolating. It would be a different story today, where slightly over half of enrollees are women.

Starting at around the time that major Supreme Court cases expanded access to birth control for women nationwide, the number of women earning advanced professional degrees—in fields like medicine, dentistry, and law—also began to dramatically increase. In the 1960s, women made up less than 5 percent of first-year law students. In 1980, this had increased to about 40 percent, and by 2000 it was nearly 50 percent. Since 2010, women have outnumbered men. When Ruth Bader Ginsburg began as a student at Harvard Law School in 1957, she was one of just nine women in a class of over 500 men. If she began law school in 2019, she would be one of nearly 300 women.

The stories for medical and dental schools are the same. Women represented a tiny fraction of students before the pill, but just two decades later, by the 1980s, they were representing a significant number (though still less than half). Today, women make up half of all graduates from medical and dental schools, as well as graduate programs (though only 40 percent of business school students).

Researchers agree that the introduction of the pill helped kick-start this cultural shift, making the pursuit of professional education a possibility for women like never before.

Women and the Workforce

Attending school is important, but for most of us, schooling is a means to an end—the pathway to a career that results in a living wage. Being able to get birth control not only allowed women to delay childrearing and pursue education, it also helped them to translate that investment into paid jobs. Women with early legal access to birth control were 20 percent more likely to have professional or managerial careers like teaching and nursing; they were 60 percent more likely to be working in advanced professional occupations.

In 1960, 32 percent of women had a job. By 2013, 59 percent did. Since the 1960s, women have made up an increasing proportion of people in skilled professions, like doctors and lawyers. Researchers estimate that more than 30 percent of the increase in the proportion of women in skilled careers from 1970 to 1990 can be attributed to access to birth control.

As women stayed in school longer and got higher paying jobs, they made more money. By age fifty, women who had early legal access to birth control in their late teens were making 8 percent more than women who did not—even though they were nearly thirty years past the point that both groups could get birth control. About one third of the total wage gains that women have made since the 1960s are due to the availability of birth control. And as more women participated in the labor force, the wage gap between men and women started to close, though not nearly fast enough.

While birth control helped narrow the gender pay gap, it still very much exists and unfortunately has stalled in recent years. In 2022, American women earned about eighty-two cents for every dollar earned by men, about the same as it was two decades earlier. There is no single, simple explanation for why the gender pay gap hasn't closed. The wage gap measure looks at total earnings by men compared to total earnings by women; it doesn't compare people of different genders in identical roles. Historically, women have been more likely to work in lower-paying professions and to do more unpaid labor. Workplace discrimination has also impacted growth potential. So even though more women are going to college and participating in the labor force now than in the past, the wage gap persists. Women start their careers earning the same as their male peers but fall behind them as their careers progress.

One reason this seems to happen is parenthood. Women who have children are less likely to have paid jobs and work fewer hours if they do work, compared to women without children. Although women and men in heterosexual relationships share more household tasks (like cooking, cleaning, and laundry) today than they did in prior generations, women are still responsible for a majority of this kind of work. On the flip side, men who are fathers are more likely to have paid jobs (and work more hours) than men without children. The different experiences that parents of different genders have create a "family gap."

Employer policies like parental leave, childcare subsidies, remote work, and flexible work hours can help women who want to keep working outside of the home do so. But these benefits are more likely to be experienced by highly educated and already advantaged women.

Today, women have more birth control options than ever before, and if they want to, they can choose to use those options to delay pregnancy. Delaying pregnancy can minimize this family gap. Women who have children in their late twenties and early thirties experience a smaller loss in wages compared to women who have children earlier, since they experience more schooling and get to a further point in their careers.

More so than ever before, women have the power to decide if and when to become a parent. Knowing this can shape a young person's goals for themselves. Being confident that one can delay or avoid pregnancy may influence someone to pursue a certain type of education or career path. The knowledge that one is securely done with childrearing can influence someone to make a career change or advancement. Knowledge is power.

Changing the World

Internationally, the story is a similar one. Over the past three decades, the number of women using modern forms of birth control has grown from 467 million in 1990 to 874 million in 2021. As birth control has become more available, more women across the world have been able to choose if and when to have children. For many women, this has meant that they can pursue opportunities like school and paid work.

Between 1960 and 1990, the number of children born to women in East and Southeast Asian countries of Singapore, Hong Kong, Taiwan, and Japan went from about six to two over the course of just one generation—an incredible demographic shift in a short amount of time. The availability of birth control wasn't solely responsible for this change, but it played an important role. According to researchers, because there were fewer children born during this time, these countries also had the five fastest-growing economies in the world—a phenomenon called the Asian Economic Miracle.

Beyond the economic impact, birth control saves lives. In more resource-limited settings, children with fewer siblings and moms who have fewer babies tend to be healthier. It's estimated that if women had full access to voluntary birth control, the number of women who die during or related to pregnancy would be 75 percent lower, and the number of infants who die would be 20 percent lower worldwide.

Even though more women are able to get birth control than ever before, access hasn't kept up with demand. Between 1990 and 2021, the number of women with an unmet need[1] for birth control grew from 147 million to 164 million women worldwide.

How Do We Measure Success?

When the pill launched in the 1960s, it's not an overstatement to say that it revolutionized the world—for women, obviously, but also for society as a whole. Birth control opened up options for women. Women began to pursue higher education and get paid jobs like never before. And today, women continue to be able to use birth control to help them achieve their economic goals. Societies have benefited from the fact that women have had these options. Women have contributed to science, politics, humanities, and the arts; they have been and will continue to be leaders.

That said, economic measures of success, like educational attainment, labor force participation, and wages, are hardly the be all and end all. They tell us something about how fair, equitable, and supportive a society is, but they certainly don't tell us everything.

For one, not everyone experienced the economic impact of birth control the same way. That was true when the pill was introduced in the United States, and it's still true. Black women, people of color, and people who are LGBTQIA+ have not benefited from the availability of birth control in the same ways as white women. Remember that forced sterilizations and reduced sentencing agreements for Norplant were happening at the very same time as these economic advancements for women in the 1960s through the 1980s. While women on average make eighty-two cents for every dollar a white man makes, the pay gap is even larger for Black women, who earn seventy cents for every dollar earned by white men, and Hispanic women, who earn sixty-five cents.

A major criticism of the world of birth control is that, up until recently, much of the discussion about how successful birth control has been in changing the world has centered on its impact on poverty. Many studies have drawn a connection between being able to get birth control and being less likely to live in poverty—both for the women using birth control and their children. This narrative has its roots in the 1960s and 1970s with the onset of publicly funded family planning. Publicly funded birth control was conceived as a tool to deal with the population crisis, and not so subtly reduce the number of babies born to lower-income families who were more likely to be Black and brown. Framing birth control as a poverty reduction approach is troublingly close to the eugenicist roots that were part of the foundation of birth control's rise to popularity.

It's also problematic because birth control can't cure poverty. To do that, we need a broad set of economic policies that help people get an affordable education, jobs with livable wages, and job advancement and growth opportunities. These are strategies like paid family leave, universal childcare, investments in public education, clean air and water, and reducing juvenile detention and incarceration that benefit everyone, especially children of color, breaking the cycle of intergenerational poverty.

Given all that, there's growing agreement that we should measure the extent to which women can get birth control when they want it, and whether birth control is meeting their needs, whatever they may be.

In the past two decades, we've seen more women in the United States able to get the birth control that they want. The Affordable Care Act eliminated out-of-pocket expenses for many women, making birth control free for the first time ever. New, highly effective methods that are now available—like the IUD and implant—have also given more options to women who want a highly effective method, as well as greater confidence that they can achieve their reproductive goals. At the same time, we know that many women still face huge obstacles when it comes to getting the birth control that they want. There is still a lot more work to be done.

Being able to get birth control when you want it is one measure of success. But what if the menu of options just isn't working for you? What if you can *get* birth control, but you just don't feel like any of the methods are what you need or want? What then? Well, I'm here to tell you that there are several new, exciting methods in the pipeline—so try not to give up hope just yet.

Remember

- **Birth control helps people choose if and when to have children.** After the pill was introduced in the United States, people had fewer babies.
- **The introduction of the birth control pill in the United States resulted in more women going to college, getting professional degrees, getting paid jobs, and earning higher wages.** Internationally, the story is similar.
- **Not everyone experienced the benefits of the introduction of the birth control pill in the same way.**
- While economic measures are important, **we should care about the extent to which women can get birth control when they want it, and whether birth control is meeting their needs.**

12

On the Cutting Edge

What the Future Holds for Birth Control

The reality is, some people are unhappy with their birth control. One in three women who have tried the pill or IUD have stopped using it because they were unsatisfied—and birth control side effects are the main reason why. Stopping a method or switching to a different method isn't inherently a bad thing. But when it's happening because women are dissatisfied with the menu of birth control options, well then that *is* a bad thing.

Surveys have shown that women are looking for more methods that last a long time (beyond the IUD and implant). They're looking for options that don't require a procedure or a visit to a clinic and that they can control themselves, keeping private from their partners or their communities. There's also a huge need for better methods to prevent the spread of STIs. The condom has basically not changed in mechanism for a hundred years—still using the same approach to STI prevention as King Minos and King Tut did.

That's not to say there hasn't been innovation in birth control. Change is the only constant in life, as they say, and birth control is no exception. In the past two decades, several new methods have been added to the menu, including the vaginal ring that lasts for twelve months; a new vaginal gel (Phexxi) that doesn't increase the risk of STIs like other spermicides do; a one-rod implant; and several new IUDs with new doses of hormones and different sizes to meet various people's needs. We not only have new methods but also new ways to get those methods. Just in 2024, the birth control pill became available over the counter for the first time.

With all the progress we've made, we still have a long way to go in meeting the pregnancy prevention needs of individuals and couples. Because of the drawbacks of existing methods, using birth control consistently and correctly can be hard. And when behaviors are hard to do, they don't happen, even when we want to do them. Think about exercise. Most of us want to do more of it, but making it happen can be difficult. Using birth control should be painless, easy—like checking your phone (which most of us *do* find the time for).

So, how do we get better birth control methods? In 1993, Congress passed a law to establish and fund research centers that are explicitly charged with pursuing and evaluating new birth control products. The National Institute of Child Health and Human Development manages this funding and tracks randomized controlled trials and related research projects.

Internationally, the Population Council's International Committee for Contraception Research brings together clinical scientists and medical professionals to identify and test new ideas for birth control. It's been through this network that such methods as the copper IUD (ParaGard®), the only nonhormonal IUD currently available, and the one-year vaginal ring (Annovera®) were developed. The

Population Council is also working on the skin gel designed for men (Nestorone®/Testosterone).

As is often the case, funding doesn't match the demand, and this is especially true in low- and middle-income countries where as many as 150 million women want birth control but can't get it. In 2018, investment in contraceptive technology in low- and middle-income countries was $64 million. There was more than twenty times as much money—$1.4 billion—invested in research and development for HIV/AIDS in these same countries.

But with that limited funding, researchers are doing the best they can to develop new and improved methods, such as those with fewer side effects for men. One area where there is a lot of work happening is developing better methods to prevent both pregnancy and STIs. Let's take a look at those promising methods first.

On the Horizon: Simultaneous Prevention of Pregnancy and STIs

A single method that prevents pregnancy and STIs has the potential to be a huge game changer. Why? Remember that on top of the need for better pregnancy prevention products, there is an epidemic of STIs happening in the United States, *and* STIs are becoming resistant to antibiotics, which makes them harder to treat. Currently, the only "multipurpose prevention technology" (i.e., a product that prevents both STIs and pregnancy) is the condom, which has its benefits but also many drawbacks, which lead to inconsistent and incorrect use. Researchers are currently exploring different approaches.

This isn't the first time that researchers have tried to create a new "multipurpose prevention technology," by the way. In the 1960s, a vaginal spermicide Nonoxynol-9 ("N-9") was introduced. At first, it seemed like this spermicide might be doubly effective at preventing pregnancy and STIs by killing off both sperm and STIs before they could be transmitted. Unfortunately, this turned out to be disastrously incorrect, as N-9 spermicide not only was ineffective at preventing HIV but actually *increased* the risk of transmission. This is why we study these things closely!

But the promise of a vaginal gel that could both prevent pregnancy and STIs lived on, and researchers are continuing to explore this option. The vaginal gel, Phexxi, has been approved by the FDA since 2020. It is currently only available with a prescription and is only approved for pregnancy prevention, but one study showed that Phexxi reduced the risk of chlamydia by 50 percent and of gonorrhea by 80 percent—a promising result.

Another promising idea is a single pill that can prevent both STIs and pregnancy. Already on the market is a pill that prevents HIV (called "pre-exposure prophylaxis" or PrEP). Researchers are attempting to combine the ingredients in PrEP with birth control pills for dual prevention. It's not a huge leap to consider how other types of birth control, like the vaginal ring, patch, or shot, could also be combined with HIV prevention drugs.

The Population Council is also working on a "fast-dissolving insert" or FDI. The FDI is small and placed inside the vagina at or around the time of sex. It quickly dissolves and starts working. The developers are testing how well it prevents pregnancy, HIV, and other STIs. The benefit of the FDI is that someone can take it right before sex, letting them keep complete control over when (and when not) to use it.

The hope is that by combining pregnancy prevention and STI prevention, people who are more motivated to prevent one will have the added benefit of preventing another outcome. Surveys suggest that people would be more interested in taking a product that prevents both STIs and pregnancy, versus a product that prevents only one.

A Better Mousetrap: New and Improved Versions of Current Methods

Researchers are looking for ways to improve upon methods that we already have. Because side effects are the main reason that people stop using birth control, researchers are trying to make side effects better. They are testing lower doses of hormones, developing new formulations of hormones, and exploring more progestin-only methods for people who can't or don't want to take estrogen. For example, a progestin-only ring or patch would complement the versions we currently have, both of which have estrogen.

Researchers are also exploring how to make current methods last longer. This is what happened with the Annovera vaginal ring, which was approved in 2018. For about fifteen years before that, the only vaginal ring on the market was a monthly ring (NuvaRing), which had to be replaced each month. The Annovera ring, developed by the Population Council, lasts for a year; the same ring is placed in the vagina for three weeks and then removed for a week for twelve consecutive months. People using Annovera don't need to make a monthly trip to a pharmacy, and they also don't need to store Annovera in the fridge, as was the case with NuvaRing (another bonus).

In a similar way, researchers are exploring how to make a once-a-month pill. Remembering to take a pill every day can be challenging, but a lot of people really like the idea of taking a pill for birth control. Researchers are working on a pill that slowly releases hormones evenly over a month (this is much trickier to do than it might sound). For women who like the shot, researchers are also working on a version that lasts for six months, doubling the length of the currently available shot (three months) and effectively cutting the number of shots someone has to get in half. The possible drawback of this is that the person is "stuck" with the method until the course of the injection runs out, as it's impossible to withdraw the hormones once they're injected. Someone wouldn't be able to immediately stop the method and would have to wait until the hormones left the body's systems first.

There's also work being done to make better nonhormonal methods. Researchers are exploring how to use different materials and designs to improve the experience of using condoms, diaphragms, and nonhormonal IUDs. Researchers are also working on expanding the menu of nonhormonal options. For example, one new method in development is a nonhormonal vaginal ring that has a mesh barrier that physically blocks and immobilizes sperm.

The Stuff of Science Fiction

Beyond trying to enhance what we currently have, researchers are also working on developing entirely new approaches to birth control. Some of these methods sound like they belong in a futuristic sci-fi movie.

One new method in development is called a micro-array patch (also called microneedle, but understandably this comes with some branding challenges). It is kind of like a bandage that sticks onto the skin, similar to the currently available birth control patch. But unlike the patch, the bandage is then removed from the skin, leaving behind tiny little projections that dissolve and release hormones into the body over an extended period of time. The benefits of this new approach are that it's simple to use, can be done at home, can be kept hidden (much more so than the currently available patch, which remains on the skin), and also doesn't have the same risk that the current patch has of accidentally falling off the skin.

There's also work being done to develop more eco-friendly approaches. Some of this relates to *how* methods are developed, reducing the environmental footprint of the manufacturing, packaging, transportation, and supply chain systems. Researchers are also working on a biodegradable contraceptive implant. Casea S is currently in clinical trials and lasts for up to two years before dissolving. This would eliminate the requirement for someone to return to a healthcare provider to have the implant removed.

Researchers are exploring different strategies for "on-demand" birth control, that is, birth control that can be taken immediately before or around the time of sex. The currently available on-demand methods are barrier methods (condoms and diaphragm) and spermicides. The "fast-dissolving insert" that is being tested for pregnancy and STI prevention is one new "on-demand" method. Other researchers are working on a thin topical film (think something like a Listerine strip) that goes inside the vagina and quickly dissolves, releasing substances that prevent pregnancy. Theoretically, this film could also be designed to prevent STIs too. Such methods are likely to be inexpensive and easy to hide, and have minimal side effects.

One research team is working on a project to use 3D printing to create personalized IUDs. The idea is that personalized IUDs would cause less discomfort during insertion and have fewer side effects. 3D printing also presents other opportunities; for example, it's also been used to develop a drug-filled vaginal ring used to treat vaginal infections and menopause symptoms. We're still a long way off from this, though.

Tubal ligation—known colloquially as getting one's tubes tied—is among the most common forms of birth control. Being a surgical procedure, sterilization is quite complicated. Surgery can be especially challenging in low-resource settings. Picture an operating room and all of the tools, materials, supplies, and staff that are required to make an operation go smoothly. Now picture that *and* you're in a really rural place. So researchers are trying to develop sterilization approaches that don't require surgery. One idea is to develop a foam that would be inserted into the cervix. Whatever permanent methods are tried, the need for appropriate counseling and informed consent remains essential.

To get really sci-fi on you, there's also work being done to explore a birth control microchip that would be inserted into the body. The person would have the ability to turn on and off the hormones using a remote. Someone could turn off the birth control when trying to get pregnant or simply during a period of abstinence. They could turn it back on when ready to start having sex. The device could last as long as sixteen years. Obviously, this approach raises some questions and concerns. Would people be comfortable having a microchip? Such a device could place someone at increased risk for reproductive coercion (if a partner were, for example, to take control of the remote). On the other hand, this might make long-term birth control more appealing to someone knowing that they could start and stop birth control without having to go back to a health care provider.

So . . . When Can I Get One?

There's a lot of work happening to expand the menu of birth control options: to give users more control over their birth control, to make methods with fewer side effects, to provide other benefits like dual pregnancy and STI prevention. The idea is to complement, not replace, our existing methods. An expanded menu helps everyone and would include more and better options for men. There are as many preferences as there are people, and having more options will only increase the chances that anyone can find a method that works best for their needs and preferences. Even though preferences and needs will likely change over time, more options mean more directions a person can take.

Maybe one of these new methods sounds intriguing to you. Maybe they all sound a little too new. They definitely all need more testing and evaluation. However you're feeling about it, know that it will be a long way off before these methods come to market; my guess is that many of them won't even make it that far.

Many methods currently under development will fail to make it through the drug and medical device development processes. Remember that this process is very expensive. Even before researchers can start testing in people, they have to prove that methods are safe and effective. In 2019, the FDA said they expect researchers studying birth control methods to submit data on 20,000 menstrual cycles (the equivalent of 1,500 person-years) on at least 400 enrolled couples for at least a year. Many development initiatives simply run out of funding or fail to show compelling enough results to continue.

Because the development process is so expensive (and because there were a number of low-cost methods already available), major pharmaceutical companies stopped developing new birth control methods in the early 2000s. Funders like the US government (National Institutes of Health and US Agency for International Development), private foundations (like the Bill and Melinda Gates Foundation), and private donors are trying to fill the gap.

Private foundations and donors have long played a crucial role in funding birth control research. Remember Katharine McCormick who funded the research to develop the birth control pill? Besides the Bill and Melinda Gates Foundation, one of the most prominent donors today is the Susan Thompson Buffett Foundation, named for the late wife of billionaire investor Warren Buffett. While it can feel disconcerting that just a few people can push the agenda on an issue as personal as reproductive health, without the philanthropic support they provide, millions of people around the world wouldn't have birth control.

More recently, pharmaceutical companies are rejoining the market. Bayer and Organon, for example, established agreements with small biotech companies doing innovative research and development. One can hope that this is a sign of renewed commitment to investing in strategies to meet the unmet demand for better birth control options.

In the meantime, before we have a menu of hundreds of birth control options to choose from, we can—really we must—do a better job of making it easier for people who want birth control to get the options that we *do* have.

Remember

- **Using birth control correctly and consistently should be easy to do for people who want to prevent pregnancy.**
- **Researchers are working on new and improved birth control methods** that simultaneously protect against pregnancy and STIs; have fewer side effects; last longer; and give people more control.
- **Funding for new methods is largely coming from the US government and private foundations and donors.**

13

Birth Control Needs You

Given all the benefits that birth control can offer—from achieving one's reproductive goals, to treating conditions and managing pain, to preventing STIs—it is all the more frustrating to see obstacles that make it harder for people to get birth control when they want it.

While the Affordable Care Act extended health insurance and eliminated the cost of birth control for many people, its political dismantling has meant that those benefits didn't get extended to everyone. Eight percent of Americans are still without health insurance; meanwhile, American Indian, Alaska Native, and Hispanic people are almost twice as likely to be uninsured. The affordability of birth control remains a concern for many people. And although the Title X Family Planning Program provides reproductive health care regardless of someone's insurance or income, it continues to be funded at the same level it was in 2005, despite the fact that demand and costs have increased during that time. Beyond cost, childcare, work, and transportation can make it hard to get birth control. And regrettably, we still have a long way to go to repair the effects of racism in reproductive health care that have led to mistrust and avoidance of the health care system.

Recently, we've seen laws being proposed and some passed that either overtly exclude birth control—like those that don't reimburse for certain types of methods—or can be misinterpreted in a way that threatens the availability of birth control, especially emergency contraception like Plan B and IUDs. We've already seen how these policies can shut down access to services like IVF and emergency contraception. And while so far those shutdowns have been temporary, that should not let us breathe easily.

Yet just 21 percent of Americans think the right to birth control is threatened.

This Is Where I Leave You

How is it that attacks on birth control continue? Because we allow them to happen. Because we don't talk about birth control nearly enough for how much of an impact it makes in our day-to-day lives. Why is that?

Perhaps it is because we have been led to believe that birth control is controversial. But there is widespread support for birth control. Nearly all voters (96 percent) think women should be able to get birth control. Over 99 percent of sexually experienced US women between the ages of fifteen to forty-four have ever used birth control, and at any given time 80–90 percent of women are using birth control—a number that is fairly consistent across race, marital status, income level, age, sexual orientation, and insurance status. Even across religious affiliations, the vast majority of people are using birth control. Birth control might be a lot of things, but controversial ain't one of them.

Maybe we accept the attacks on birth control because we feel uneducated, like we're not equipped enough to engage in discussions about what birth control is and why we need it. But birth control is important to us; 74 percent of women say that preventing pregnancy is important. For something so important to our lives, it deserves to have our support. By reading this book, I hope you've learned a few things you didn't know about birth control.

Perhaps we're willing to sit back and watch attacks on birth control because to talk about it would involve talking about taboo topics. Sex, for one. Talking about sex makes us weirdly uncomfortable, given how common it is. But also the noncontraceptive benefits of birth control bring up other topics we don't like to discuss: gynecological conditions, diseases that are transmitted through sex, cancer. But if we let our fear of talking about these subjects prevent us from being willing to speak up, we risk not having the option to talk about these topics at all. If talking about it is hard, then hopefully reading about it is easier. But reading about it won't be enough.

Now that you are done with this book, I have two requests for you. First, I hope you believe that you deserve to find a birth control strategy that works for you—and yes, that might be no birth control at all. There is no perfect method, and there are pros and cons to all of the methods out there (with some on the horizon that seek to address those drawbacks), but everyone deserves a strategy that meets their needs and preferences. And I'll say it again: Everyone deserves support from a healthcare provider to make that happen.

The second request is to refuse to sit quietly and watch attacks on birth control happen. We can't assume that the right to birth control is secure. Policies that restrict our ability to get birth control will be harmful. It's time to use our vote, our voice, and our power to make it clear that these policies take away our basic rights—they are not what we want. To that end, I need you to become more comfortable talking about birth control and to share what you learned from this book with your friends, families, neighbors, and colleagues. I will leave you with five key messages to help make this communication easier. I am counting on you to be an advocate for birth control so that everyone, everywhere, can create the families that they want.

Five Key Messages about Birth Control to Tell your Friends and Family

1. In the words of the collective of Black women who developed the concept of reproductive justice, **everyone has the right to have and not have children and to make decisions about their own bodies.** Birth control can help people do that.
2. **Birth control is widely used and nearly universally accepted.** Almost everyone uses birth control across demographic, geographic, political, and religious lines. And nearly everyone agrees that people should be able to get birth control when they want it.
3. **The menu of birth control options is large and growing.** There are lots of reasons why people use birth control: pregnancy prevention, treatment of medical conditions, and prevention of STIs. Each person should decide for themselves which method is right for them based on what's important to them and which they'll use correctly and consistently. There are new methods being developed for men and women.
4. **Birth control has helped make our society more equal.** When birth control became available in the United States, it helped women obtain more education, participate more in the labor force, and earn higher wages. Not everyone experienced these benefits in the same way—and there's still a lot more work to be done.
5. **We all have a role to play in protecting birth control.** Laws that erroneously jeopardize emergency contraception, IUDs, or other birth control methods, threaten our ability to get birth control when we need it. Use your vote, fact-check your content, and speak up for birth control.

Keep the Discussion Going

Book Club Questions

1. What was the most interesting chapter you read, and why?
2. How has birth control changed over its existence? What did you see as some of the most defining points in birth control's history?
3. What aspects of the history of birth control were surprising to you?
4. Birth control is often portrayed as controversial and divisive. What factors have contributed to this understanding?
5. When considering the future of birth control, what do you find most exciting? What are you concerned about?
6. How does what you read make you rethink what birth control means for your own life?
7. How does what you read make you rethink what birth control means for the world?

Tools and Resources

These resources are great for exploring and comparing birth control methods:

- Bedsider: https://www.bedsider.org/birth-control
- Planned Parenthood: https://www.plannedparenthood.org/learn/birth-control
- The University of California, San Francisco, "My Birth Control" https://use.mybirthcontrol.org/

Complementary Reading

- *A Good Time to Be Born: How Science and Public Health Gave Children a Future* by Perri Klass, MD
- *Killing the Black Body: Race, Reproduction, and the Meaning of Liberty* by Dorothy Roberts, JD
- *The Immortal Life of Henrietta Lacks* by Rebecca Skloot
- *Lady Tan's Circle of Women* by Lisa See
- *Legacy: A Black Physician Reckons with Racism in Medicine* by Uché Blackstock, MD
- *Strange Bedfellows: Adventures in the Science, History, and Surprising Secrets of STDs* by Ina Park, MD
- *Take My Hand* by Dolen Perkins-Valdez, PhD

Acknowledgments

Thank you to those who made this book happen: my agent, Anne Devlin, as well as the editing and production team of Jacquie Flynn, Mikayla Lindsay, and many others at Bloomsbury.

Thank you to the early readers who made the book better, especially Jaya Mathur, Frances Marshman, Jennifer Kawatu, Liza Boffi, Francesca Cocuzza, and McKenzie LaRouere.

Thank you to my motivators: my parents for setting a high bar, my husband for enduring patience and support, and my boys for giving me hope for the future.

And finally, the greatest of thanks to the tens of thousands of professionals who provide birth control and other essential reproductive health care in the United States and around the world. We need you.

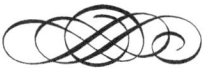

Notes

Introduction

1. In this book I generally use "women" to refer to people with the potential ability to become pregnant, and "men" to refer to people who have the potential ability to cause pregnancy. My intention is not to exclude anyone for whom this is not the case, and I have tried to incorporate a wide range of experiences about birth control throughout this book.

Chapter 1

1. By the way, there may be something to the hypothesis that pomegranate seeds are fertility enhancing. There are researchers still exploring that question. But there is definitely no reason to use a pomegranate rind for birth control any more. We have much, much better options than that.

2. Some "grandfathered" plans and health plans sponsored by certain organizations that have a religious objection don't have to cover contraceptive methods and counseling.

Chapter 2

1. A fancy word for strong sexual desire. Count on clergymen to find a way to make sexual desire sound so…unsexy.

2   This data is from two different polls. The poll of all Americans was conducted in 2022. The poll looking at the data by Christian denomination was conducted in 2016.

Chapter 3

1   We actually face a very different picture of population growth today. Today, the rate of population growth is about half of what it was when it peaked in 1962. By 2050, over three-quarters (155 of 204) of countries will not have high enough fertility rates to sustain population size. By 2100, this is expected to increase to 97% of countries (198 of 204).

Chapter 5

1   Technically there are actually many different versions of the pill containing different types and dosages of hormones, but in practice we just lump them all together as "the pill."

Chapter 6

1   No affiliation with Birthright Israel that supports young Jewish people to travel to Israel.

Chapter 7

1   For more on this, read *Killing the Black Body: Race, Reproduction, and the Meaning of Liberty* by Dorothy Roberts.

Chapter 9

1   There are two accepted measures of birth control effectiveness: a "perfect use" rate assumes the method is used consistently and correctly every time,

whereas a "typical use" rate is the level of effectiveness in real-world settings, taking into account that methods are not used consistently and correctly 100% of the time. This section reports typical use rates.

2. Prior to 2006, a prescription was needed for Plan B. Beginning in 2016, Plan B and generic equivalents were made available without a prescription for people 17 and older. In 2014, the FDA removed the age requirements such that now Plan B (and generic equivalents) can be bought over the counter at any age.

Chapter 10

1. LGBTQIA+ stands for lesbian, gay, bisexual, transgender, queer, intersex, asexual, and other identities
2. For a great, funny read about STIs, check out *Strange Bedfellows: Adventures in the Science, History, and Surprising Secrets of STDs* by Ina Park
3. This measure excludes married people.

Chapter 11

1. The United Nations defines women who are capable of becoming pregnant and sexually active who wish to stop or delay childbearing but are not using any form of contraception as having "unmet need" for birth control. (Women who are pregnant at the time of data collection and report that the pregnancy was unwanted or mistimed are also included in this "unmet need" category.)

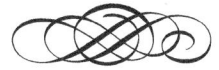

References

Introduction

"Abortion Laws by State - Center for Reproductive Rights," *Center for Reproductive Rights*, May 7, 2024. https://reproductiverights.org/maps/abortion-laws-by-state/.

"ART Success Rates | CDC," n.d. https://www.cdc.gov/art/artdata/index.html.

"Dobbs V. Jackson Women's Health Organization (2022)," LII / Legal Information Institute, *Cornell Law School*, March 15, 2024. https://www.law.cornell.edu/wex/dobbs_v._jackson_women%27s_health_organization_%282022%29#.

Felix, Mabel Laurie Sobel, and Alina Salganicoff. "The Right to Contraception: State and Federal Actions, Misinformation, and the Courts," *KFF*, May 28, 2024, https://www.kff.org/womens-health-policy/issue-brief/the-right-to-contraception-state-and-federal-actions-misinformation-and-the-courts/.

Guttmacher Institute. "Contraceptive Use in the United States by Demographics," *Guttmacher Institute*, August 24, 2022. https://www.guttmacher.org/fact-sheet/contraceptive-use-united-states.

Frederiksen, Brittni, Usha Ranji, Alina Salganicoff, and Michelle Long. "Women's Sexual and Reproductive Health Services: Key Findings From the 2020 KFF Women's Health Survey," *KFF*, April 21, 2021. https://www.kff.org/womens-health-policy/issue-brief/womens-sexual-and-reproductive-health-services-key-findings-from-the-2020-kff-womens-health-survey/.

Frederiksen, Brittni, Usha Ranji, Michelle Long, Karen Diep, and Alina Salganicoff. "Contraception in the United States: A Closer Look at Experiences, Preferences, and Coverage," *KFF*, November 18, 2022. https://www.kff.org/womens-health-policy/report/contraception-in-the-united-states-a-closer-look-at-experiences-preferences-and-coverage/.

Gale, William, and Donald Marron, "Five Myths About the 47 Percent," *Washington Post*, September 21, 2012, https://www.urban.org/sites/default/files/publication/26506/901527-Five-Myths-About-the-Percent.pdf.

Justia Law. "Dobbs V. Jackson Women's Health Organization, 597 U.S. (2022),"
Justia n.d. https://supreme.justia.com/cases/federal/us/597/19-1392/.

Kavanaugh, Megan L., Rubina Hussain, and Ashley C. Little. "Unfulfilled and Method-specific Contraceptive Preferences Among Reproductive-aged Contraceptive Users in Arizona, Iowa, New Jersey, and Wisconsin," *Health Services Research* 59, no. 3 (March 8, 2024): e1429. https://doi.org/10.1111/1475-6773.14297.

Male Contraceptive Initiative. "Interest Among U.S. Men for New Male Contraceptive Options Consumer Research Study," *MCI*, February 2019, https://www.malecontraceptive.org/uploads/1/3/1/9/131958006/mci_consumerresearchstudy.pdf.

Mascarenhas, Lauren, and Isabel Rosales, "Alabama Clinics Resume Treatment under New Ivf Law, But Experts Say It Will Take More Work to Protect Fertility Services," *CNN*, March 7, 2024.

Musa, Amanda and Isabel Rosales, "'My Journey Ends': Without Ivf, This Alabama Uterine Transplant Patient Loses Her Hope for a Second Baby," *CNN*, March 2, 2024.

National Survey of Family Growth. "NSFG - Listing C - Key Statistics From the National Survey of Family Growth," *National Center for Health Statistics* (NCHS), n.d. https://www.cdc.gov/nchs/nsfg/key_statistics/c-keystat.htm#contraception.

PerryUndem Research/Communication. "Views on Birth Control Report," n.d. https://view.publitas.com/perryundem-research-communication/views-on-birth-control-report-pdf/page/1.

Rosales, Isabel, Lauren Mascarenhas, and Chris Youd, "This Couple Has to Leave Alabama or Risk Losing Their Eggs after State Ruling Forces Providers to Pause Ivf Treatment," *CNN*, February 22, 2024.

Sharfstein, Joshua. "The Alabama Supreme Court's Ruling on Frozen Embryos," *Johns Hopkins Bloomberg School of Public Health*, February 27, 2024. https://publichealth.jhu.edu/2024/the-alabama-supreme-courts-ruling-on-frozen-embryos.

United Nations. "World Family Planning 2022," *Department of Economic and Social Affairs, Population Division*. New York, 2022. https://www.un.org/development/desa/pd/sites/www.un.org.development.desa.pd/files/files/documents/2023/Feb/undesa_pd_2022_world-family-planning.pdf.

U.S. Food and Drug Administration, "Plan B One-Step (1.5 mg levonorgestrel) Information," *FDA*. https://www.fda.gov/drugs/postmarket-drug-safety-information-patients-and-providers/plan-b-one-step-15-mg-levonorgestrel-information.

Chapter 1

Ajayi, Anthony Idowu, Oladele Vincent Adeniyi, and Wilson Akpan. "Use of Traditional and Modern Contraceptives Among Childbearing Women: Findings From a Mixed Methods Study in Two Southwestern Nigerian States," *BMC Public Health* 18, no. 1 (May 9, 2018): 604. https://doi.org/10.1186/s12889-018-5522-6.

Amy, Jean-Jacques, and Michel Thiery. "The Condom: A Turbulent History," *The European Journal of Contraception & Reproductive Health Care* 20, no. 5 (June 11, 2015): 387–402. https://doi.org/10.3109/13625187.2015.1050716.

Bhatt, Narendra, and Manasi Deshpande. "A Critical Review and Scientific Prospective on Contraceptive Therapeutics From Ayurveda and Allied Ancient Knowledge," *Frontiers in Pharmacology* 12 (June 3, 2021): 629591. https://doi.org/10.3389/fphar.2021.629591.

BrandeisNOW. "Mothers' Lives in Ancient Greece Were Not Easy – but Celebrations of Their Love Have Survived Across the Centuries," *BrandeisNOW*, n.d. https://www.brandeis.edu/now/2023/may/mothers-day.html.

Cartwright, Mark, and Marie-Lan Nguyen. "Persephone," *World History Encyclopedia*, March 29, 2023. https://www.worldhistory.org/persephone/.

Frank-Herrmann, P., J. Heil, C. Gnoth, E. Toledo, S. Baur, C. Pyper, E. Jenetzky, T. Strowitzki, and G. Freundl. "The Effectiveness of a Fertility Awareness Based Method to Avoid Pregnancy in Relation to a Couple's Sexual Behaviour During the Fertile Time: A Prospective Longitudinal Study," *Human Reproduction* 22, no. 5 (February 20, 2007): 1310–19. https://doi.org/10.1093/humrep/dem003.

Frederiksen, Brittni, Usha Ranji, Michelle Long, Karen Diep, and Alina Salganicoff. "Contraception in the United States: A Closer Look at Experiences, Preferences, and Coverage," *KFF*, November 18, 2022. https://www.kff.org/womens-health-policy/report/contraception-in-the-united-states-a-closer-look-at-experiences-preferences-and-coverage/

Gorvett, Zaria. "The Mystery of the Lost Roman Herb," *BBC*, February 24, 2022. https://www.bbc.com/future/article/20170907-the-mystery-of-the-lost-roman-herb.

Guttmacher Institute. "The Federal Contraceptive Coverage Guarantee: An Effective Policy That Should be Strengthened and Expanded," *Guttmacher*, February 20, 2024. https://www.guttmacher.org/fact-sheet/contraceptive-coverage-guarantee.

Guzzo, Karen Benjamin, and Sarah R. Hayford. "Adolescent Reproductive and Contraceptive Knowledge and Attitudes and Adult Contraceptive Behavior,"

Maternal and Child Health Journal 22, no. 1 (July 28, 2017): 32–40. https://doi.org/10.1007/s10995-017-2351-7.

Harris, Emily. "US Maternal Mortality Continues to Worsen," *JAMA* 329, no. 15 (April 18, 2023): 1248. https://doi.org/10.1001/jama.2023.5254.

Haynes, Meagan Campol, Nessa Ryan, Mona Saleh, Abigail Ford Winkel, and Veronica Ades. "Contraceptive Knowledge Assessment: Validity and Reliability of a Novel Contraceptive Research Tool," *Contraception* 95, no. 2 (February 1, 2017): 190–97. https://doi.org/10.1016/j.contraception.2016.09.002.

HealthCare.gov. "Birth Control Benefits and Reproductive Health Care Options in the Health Insurance Marketplace," *Healthcare*, n.d. https://www.healthcare.gov/coverage/birth-control-benefits/.

Hill, Latoya, Samantha Artiga, and Usha Ranji. "Racial Disparities in Maternal and Infant Health: Current Status and Efforts to Address Them," *KFF*, June 15, 2023. https://www.kff.org/racial-equity-and-health-policy/issue-brief/racial-disparities-in-maternal-and-infant-health-current-status-and-efforts-to-address-them/.

Jang, Caleb, and Henry Lee. "A Review of Racial Disparities in Infant Mortality in the US," *Children* 9, no. 2 (February 14, 2022): 257. https://doi.org/10.3390/children9020257.

Justia Law. "Burwell V. Hobby Lobby Stores, Inc., 573 U.S. 682 (2014)," n.d. https://supreme.justia.com/cases/federal/us/573/682/.

Khalil, Rami Bou, and Sami Richa. "When Affective Disorders Were Considered to Emanate from the Heart: The Ebers Papyrus," *The American Journal of Psychiatry* 171, no. 3 (March 1, 2014): 275. https://doi.org/10.1176/appi.ajp.2013.13070860.

Khan, Md Nuruzzaman, and Shimlin Jahan Khanam. "The Effectiveness of WHO's Interpregnancy Interval Advice," *The Lancet Global Health* 11, no. 10 (October 1, 2023): e1476–77. https://doi.org/10.1016/s2214-109x(23)00402-3.

Knowles, Jon, et al. "A History of Birth Control Methods," *Planned Parenthood Federation of America*, 2012. https://www.plannedparenthood.org/files/2613/9611/6275/History_of_BC_Methods.pdf.

"Lactational Amenorrhea Method," *Access Esperanza Clinics*, n.d. https://accessclinics.org/birthcontrol/lactational-amenorrhea-method-lam/

"Lactational Amenorrhea Method – USMEC," *CDC*, n.d. https://www.cdc.gov/reproductivehealth/contraception/mmwr/mec/appendixg.html.

Lopes, Helena Trindade, and Ronaldo G. Gurgel Pereira. "The Gynaecological Papyrus Kahun," *CDN*. https://cdn.intechopen.com/pdfs/78710.pdf

Lowder, J. Bryan. "When Did Humans Realize That Sex Leads to Pregnancy?" *Slate Magazine*, January 10, 2013. https://slate.com/technology/2013/01/

when-did-humans-realize-sex-makes-babies-evolution-of-reproductive-consciousness-of-the-cause-of-pregnancy.html.

Melbostad, Heidi S., Gary J. Badger, Catalina N. Rey, Lauren K. MacAfee, Anne K. Dougherty, Stacey C. Sigmon, and Sarah H. Heil. "Contraceptive Knowledge Among Females and Males Receiving Medication Treatment for Opioid Use Disorder Compared to Those Seeking Primary Care," *Substance Use & Misuse* 55, no. 14 (October 5, 2020): 2403–8. https://doi.org/10.1080/10826084.2020.1823418.

Molitoris, Joseph, Kieron Barclay, and Martin Kolk. "When and Where Birth Spacing Matters for Child Survival: An International Comparison Using the DHS," *Demography* 56, no. 4 (July 3, 2019): 1349–70. https://doi.org/10.1007/s13524-019-00798-y.

Moroole, Molelekwa A., Simeon A. Materechera, Wilfred Otang-Mbeng, and Adeyemi O. Aremu. "African Indigenous Contraception: A Review," *African Journal of Reproductive Health* 24, no. 4 (December 1, 2020): 173–84. https://doi.org/10.29063/ajrh2020/v24i4.18.

Nikseresht, Mohsen, Ali Reza Fallahzadeh, Mehdi Akbartabar Toori, and Reza Mahmoudi. "Effects of Pomegranate Seed Oil on the Fertilization Potency of Rat's Sperm," *Journal of Clinical and Diagnostic Research*, January 1, 2015. https://doi.org/10.7860/jcdr/2015/12576.6853.

"NSFG – Listing C – Key Statistics From the National Survey of Family Growth," *CDC*, n.d. https://www.cdc.gov/nchs/nsfg/key_statistics/c-keystat.htm#contraception.

Planned Parenthood. "What Is the Cervical Mucus Method? | Cycle, Stages & Chart," n.d. https://www.plannedparenthood.org/learn/birth-control/fertility-awareness/whats-cervical-mucus-method-fams.

Quirke, Stephen. "Kahun Medical Papyrus," *University College London*, 2002 https://www.ucl.ac.uk/museums-static/digitalegypt/med/birthpapyrus.html.

Rossier, Clémentine, and Jamaica Corker. "Contemporary Use of Traditional Contraception in sub-Saharan Africa," *Population and Development Review* 43, no. S1 (January 20, 2017): 192–215. https://doi.org/10.1111/padr.12008.

Smith, Lesley. "Ancient Condoms," *Journal of Family Planning and Reproductive Health Care* 33, no. 1 (January 1, 2007): 66. https://doi.org/10.1783/147118907779399783.

Smith, Lesley. "The Kahun Gynaecological Papyrus: Ancient Egyptian Medicine," *Journal of Family Planning and Reproductive Health Care* 37, no. 1 (January 1, 2011): 54–5. https://doi.org/10.1136/jfprhc.2010.0019.

Statista. "Child Mortality in the United States 1800–2020," July 4, 2024. https://www.statista.com/statistics/1041693/united-states-all-time-child-mortality-rate/.

"Tan Yunxian – Step Inside: Lady Tan's Circle of Women," *Lisa See*, n.d. https://lisasee.com/step-inside/lady-tan-and-chinese-medicine/

Vekemans, M. "Postpartum Contraception: The Lactational Amenorrhea Method," *The European Journal of Contraception & Reproductive Health Care* 2, no. 2 (January 1, 1997): 105–11. https://doi.org/10.3109/13625189709167463.

Verghese, Abraham. "Where Do Babies Come From? And Why Did It Take Scientists So Long to Find Out?" *New York Times*, June 23, 2017.

Wessel, Gary M. "Of Camels, Silkworms, and Contraception," *Molecular Reproduction and Development* 81, no. 9 (September 1, 2014). https://doi.org/10.1002/mrd.22416.

Wills, Matthew. "The Paradoxical Pomegranate," *JSTOR Daily*, November 23, 2021. https://daily.jstor.org/the-paradoxical-pomegranate/.

Zaid, Siti Sarah Mohamad, Siti Suraya Ruslee, and Mohd Helmy Mokhtar. "Protective Roles of Honey in Reproductive Health: A Review," *Molecules* 26, no. 11 (June 1, 2021): 3322. https://doi.org/10.3390/molecules26113322.

Chapter 2

Alomair, Noura, Samah Alageel, Nathan Davies, and Julia V. Bailey. "Muslim Women's Views and Experiences of Family Planning in Saudi Arabia: A Qualitative Study," *BMC Women S Health* 23, no. 1 (November 25, 2023). https://doi.org/10.1186/s12905-023-02786-2.

Betancourt, Roland. "Abortion and Contraception in the Middle Ages," *Scientific American*, February 20, 2024. https://www.scientificamerican.com/article/abortion-and-contraception-in-the-middle-ages/.

Bible Gateway. "Genesis 1:28 (KJV)," n.d. https://www.biblegateway.com/passage/?search=Genesis%201%3A28&version=KJV.

Blazina, Carrie. "8 Key Findings About Catholics and Abortion," *Pew Research Center*, April 14, 2024. https://www.pewresearch.org/short-reads/2020/10/20/8-key-findings-about-catholics-and-abortion/.

Bose, Tulika. "The Surprising Backstory Behind Witch Hunts and Reproductive Labor," *Scientific American*, February 20, 2024. https://www.scientificamerican.com/podcast/episode/the-surprising-backstory-behind-witch-hunts-and-reproductive-labor/.

Brenan, Megan. "Americans Say Birth Control, Divorce Most 'Morally Acceptable,'" *Gallup.Com*, March 14, 2024. https://news.gallup.com/poll/393515/americans-say-birth-control-divorce-morally-acceptable.aspx.

Budhwani, Henna, Jami Anderson, and Kristine R. Hearld. "Muslim Women's Use of Contraception in the United States," *Reproductive Health* 15, no. 1 (January 5, 2018): 1. https://doi.org/10.1186/s12978-017-0439-6.

Dittrick Medical History Center. "19th Century Artifacts," n.d. https://artsci.case.edu/dittrick/online-exhibits/history-of-birth-control/contraception-in-america-1800-1900/19th-century-artifacts/.

Dittrick Medical History Center. "Anthony Comstock's Influence," n.d. https://artsci.case.edu/dittrick/online-exhibits/history-of-birth-control/contraception-in-america-1800-1900/anthony-comstocks-influence/.

Dittrick Medical History Center. "The Civil War: Sex and Soldiers," n.d. https://artsci.case.edu/dittrick/online-exhibits/history-of-birth-control/contraception-in-america-1800-1900/the-civil-war-sex-and-soldiers/.

Dittrick Medical History Center. "Douching and Spermicides," n.d. https://artsci.case.edu/dittrick/online-exhibits/history-of-birth-control/contraception-in-america-1900-1950/douching-and-spermicides/.

Dittrick Medical History Center. "Early Literature," n.d. https://artsci.case.edu/dittrick/online-exhibits/history-of-birth-control/contraception-in-america-1800-1900/early-literature/.

Drucker, Donna J. "Contraceptive Knowledge in the Mid-19th-Century United States," *Circulating Now From the NLM Historical Collections*, July 23, 2021. https://circulatingnow.nlm.nih.gov/2019/12/05/contraceptive-knowledge-in-the-mid-19th-century-united-states/.

Feldman, P. "Sexuality, Birth Control and Childbirth in Orthodox Jewish Tradition," *PubMed Central (PMC)*, January 1, 1992. https://www.ncbi.nlm.nih.gov/pmc/articles/PMC1488204/.

Francis. "Post-Synodal Apostolic Exhortation Amoris Lætitia," *Vatican*, 2016, https://www.vatican.va/content/dam/francesco/pdf/apost_exhortations/documents/papa-francesco_esortazione-ap_20160319_amoris-laetitia_en.pdf.

"The Future of the Global Muslim Population – Main Factors Driving Population Growth," *Pew Research Center*, January 27, 2011. https://www.pewresearch.org/religion/2011/01/27/future-of-the-global-muslim-population-main-factors/.

"The Future of the Global Muslim Population – Related Factors," *Pew Research Center*, January 27, 2011. https://www.pewresearch.org/religion/2011/01/27/future-of-the-global-muslim-population-related-factors/.

Gallup, Inc. "Moral Issues | Gallup Historical Trends," *Gallup.com*, July 9, 2024. https://news.gallup.com/poll/1681/Moral-Issues.aspx.

Gnanawimala. B. "Free to Choose. The Buddhist View," *Asiaweek*, October 27, 1993. https://pubmed.ncbi.nlm.nih.gov/12345273/.

Goldberg, Michelle. "Trump's Allies Say They'll Enforce the Comstock Act. Believe Them," *New York Times*, June 21 2024. https://www.nytimes.com/2024/06/21/opinion/trump-comstock-act-abortion.html

Guttmacher Institute. "People of All Religions Use Birth Control and Have Abortions," August 31, 2022. https://www.guttmacher.org/article/2020/10/people-all-religions-use-birth-control-and-have-abortions.

Hacker, J. David, and Evan Roberts. "Fertility Decline in the United States, 1850–1930: New Evidence From Complete-count Datasets," *Annales De DéMographie Historique* 138, no. 2 (April 10, 2020): 143–77. https://doi.org/10.3917/adh.138.0143.

"How Birth Control Methods Prevent Pregnancy," n.d. https://myhealth.alberta.ca/Health/Pages/conditions.aspx?hwid=tb1025.

"Humanae Vitae (July 25, 1968) | Paul VI," *Vatican*, July 24, 1968. https://www.vatican.va/content/paul-vi/en/encyclicals/documents/hf_p-vi_enc_25071968_humanae-vitae.html.

"The Impact of 25 Years of 'Humanae Vitae'," *PubMed*, August 1, 1993. https://pubmed.ncbi.nlm.nih.gov/12345157/.

Jones, Rachel K., Joerg Dreweke, and Guttmacher Institute. "Countering Conventional Wisdom: New Evidence on Religion and Contraceptive Use," edited by Haley Ball. *Guttmacher Institute*, 2011. https://www.guttmacher.org/sites/default/files/pdfs/pubs/Religion-and-Contraceptive-Use.pdf.

Knowles, Jon, et al. "A History of Birth Control Methods," *Planned Parenthood Federation of America*, 2012. https://www.plannedparenthood.org/files/2613/9611/6275/History_of_BC_Methods.pdf.

Koffman, Lori. "Jewish Perspectives on Reproductive Realities," *NCJW*, n.d. https://www.ncjw.org/wp-content/uploads/2018/02/Jewish-Perspective-on-Reproductive-Realities-FORMATTED11.pdf.

Lieberman, Hallie. "A Short History of the Condom," *JSTOR Daily*, June 21, 2018. https://daily.jstor.org/short-history-of-the-condom/.

"Newborn and Infant Breastfeeding," *American Academy of Pediatrics*, 2022. https://www.aap.org/en/patient-care/newborn-and-infant-nutrition/newborn-and-infant-breastfeeding/#.

PBS. "Anthony Comstock's 'Chastity' Laws," *American Experience*, March 13, 2018. https://www.pbs.org/wgbh/americanexperience/features/pill-anthony-comstocks-chastity-laws/.

Poggioli, Sylvia. "After 10 Years as Pope, Francis Continues to Reshape the Catholic Church," *NPR*, March 13, 2023. https://www.npr.org/2023/03/13/1162954465/after-10-years-as-pope-francis-continues-to-reshape-the-catholic-church.

Potts, Malcolm. "Birth Control | Description, History, Types, & Effectiveness," *Encyclopedia Britannica*, July 11, 2024. https://www.britannica.com/science/birth-control/Ethics-and-the-influence-of-religious-systems.

Price, David. "Mother's Friend: Birth Control in Nineteenth-Century America," *National Museum of Civil War Medicine*, March 11, 2022. https://www.civilwarmed.org/birth-control.

Rahnama, Parvin, Alireza Hidarnia, Farkhondeh Amin Shokravi, Anoushiravan Kazemnejad, Deborah Oakley, and Ali Montazeri. "Why Iranian Married Women Use Withdrawal Instead of Oral Contraceptives? A Qualitative Study From Iran," *BMC Public Health* 10, no. 1 (May 28, 2010): 289. https://doi.org/10.1186/1471-2458-10-289.

Roudi-Fahimi, Farzaneh, and Population Reference Bureau. "Islam and Family Planning," *PRB MENA Policy Brief*, 2004. https://www.prb.org/wp-content/uploads/2004/09/IslamFamilyPlanning.pdf.

Rowell, Hunter H. "'The Ethics of Marriage,'" *Journal of the American Medical Association* XI, no. 12 (September 22, 1888): 429. https://doi.org/10.1001/jama.1888.02400640033013.

Schenker, Joseph G., and Vicki Rabenou. "Contraception: Traditional and Religious Attitudes," *European Journal of Obstetrics, Gynecology, and Reproductive Biology* 49, no. 1–2 (April 1, 1993): 15–18. https://pubmed.ncbi.nlm.nih.gov/8365507/.

Srinivas, M. N. "A Part of Life. The Hindu View," *Asiaweek*, October 27, 1993. https://pubmed.ncbi.nlm.nih.gov/12345274/.

Stone, Geoffrey R. "Sex and the First Amendment: The Long and Winding History of Obscenity Law," *First Amendment Law Review, University of North Carolina*, 17: 134–46 https://scholarship.law.unc.edu/cgi/viewcontent.cgi?article=1267&context=falr.

Weisner, Caitlin. "Warts and All: Learn the Fascinating History of Witchcraft and Reproductive Health," *New York Historical Society*, October 29, 2019. https://www.nyhistory.org/blogs/witchcraft-and-reproductive-health.

Chapter 3

Abrams, Abigail. "No, Birth Control Doesn't Make You Have Riskier Sex, Researchers Say," *TIME*, October 12, 2017. https://time.com/4975951/donald-trump-birth-control-mandate-sexual-behavior/.

Atske, Sara, and Sara Atske. "Social Media Use in 2021," *Pew Research Center*, April 7, 2021. https://www.pewresearch.org/internet/2021/04/07/social-media-use-in-2021/.

Bailey, Martha J. "Fifty Years of Family Planning: New Evidence on the Long-Run Effects of Increasing Access to Contraception," *Brookings Papers on Economic Activity* 2013, no. 1 (March 1, 2013): 341–409. https://doi.org/10.1353/eca.2013.0001.

Brenan, Megan. "Religion Considered Important to 72% of Americans," *Gallup. Com*, December 24, 2018. https://news.gallup.com/poll/245651/religion-considered-important-americans.aspx.

Brody, Jane E. "Contraception for Teenagers," *New York Times*, February 19, 2018 https://www.nytimes.com/2018/02/19/well/live/contraception-for-teenagers.html

Brown, Sarah S., and Leon Eisenberg. "Socioeconomic and Cultural Influences on Contraceptive Use," *The Best Intentions – NCBI Bookshelf*, 1995. https://www.ncbi.nlm.nih.gov/books/NBK232120/.

Butler, Adrienne Stith, and Ellen Wright Clayton. "Title X Goals, Priorities, and Accomplishments," *A Review of the HHS Family Planning Program – NCBI Bookshelf*, 2009. https://www.ncbi.nlm.nih.gov/books/NBK215201/.

Chin, Helen B., Theresa Ann Sipe, Randy Elder, Shawna L. Mercer, Sajal K. Chattopadhyay, Verughese Jacob, Holly R. Wethington, et al. "The Effectiveness of Group-Based Comprehensive Risk-Reduction and Abstinence Education Interventions to Prevent or Reduce the Risk of Adolescent Pregnancy, Human Immunodeficiency Virus, and Sexually Transmitted Infections," *American Journal of Preventive Medicine* 42, no. 3 (March 1, 2012): 272–94. https://doi.org/10.1016/j.amepre.2011.11.006.

Crum, G. "Health Care Policy and the Reagan Administration: The Case of Family Planning," *Journal of Health Human Resources Administration* 12, no. 4 (1990): 524–35. https://pubmed.ncbi.nlm.nih.gov/10105516/

Gold, Rachel Benson. "The Guttmacher Report on Public Policy," *Guttmacher*, February 2001. https://www.guttmacher.org/sites/default/files/article_files/gr040105.pdf.

Gross, Terry, and Jill Lepore. "How Birth Control and Abortion Became Politicized," *NPR*, November 9, 2011. https://www.npr.org/transcripts/142097521.

Guttmacher Institute. "Abstinence-Only-Until-Marriage Programs Are Ineffective and Harmful to Young People, Expert Review Confirms," *Guttmacher Institute*, August 22, 2017. https://www.guttmacher.org/news-release/2017/abstinence-only-until-marriage-programs-are-ineffective-and-harmful-young-people.

Guttmacher Institute. "Federally Funded Abstinence-Only Programs: Harmful and Ineffective," *Guttmacher Institute*, May 2021. https://www.guttmacher.org/fact-sheet/abstinence-only-programs.

Guttmacher Institute. "The Unprecedented Expansion of the Global Gag Rule: Trampling Rights, Health and Free Speech," *Guttmacher Institute*, August 15,

2023. https://www.guttmacher.org/gpr/2020/04/unprecedented-expansion-global-gag-rule-trampling-rights-health-and-free-speech.

Hasell, Ariel, and Sedona Chinn. "The Political Influence of Lifestyle Influencers? Examining the Relationship Between Aspirational Social Media Use and Anti-Expert Attitudes and Beliefs," *Social Media + Society* 9, no. 4 (October 1, 2023). https://doi.org/10.1177/20563051231211945.

HHS Office of Population Affairs. "Title X Turns 50," n.d. https://opa.hhs.gov/grant-programs/title-x-service-grants/title-x-turns-50.

"Humanae Vitae (July 25, 1968) | Paul VI," *Vatican*, July 24, 1968. https://www.vatican.va/content/paul-vi/en/encyclicals/documents/hf_p-vi_enc_25071968_humanae-vitae.html.

Institute for Health Metrics and Evaluation. "The Lancet: Dramatic Declines in Global Fertility Rates Set to Transform Global Population Patterns by 2100," March 20, 2024. https://www.healthdata.org/news-events/newsroom/news-releases/lancet-dramatic-declines-global-fertility-rates-set-transform.

Kantor, Leslie, and Nicole Levitz. "Parents' Views on Sex Education in Schools: How Much Do Democrats and Republicans Agree?" *PloS One* 12, no. 7 (July 3, 2017): e0180250. https://doi.org/10.1371/journal.pone.0180250.

Lasher, Craig. "Once Upon a Time: The History of Republican Support for International Family Planning and Contraception," *PAI*, June 17, 2022. https://pai.org/resources/once-upon-a-time/.

Nadeem, Reem. "How U.S. Religious Composition Has Changed in Recent Decades," *Pew Research Center*, September 13, 2022. https://www.pewresearch.org/religion/2022/09/13/how-u-s-religious-composition-has-changed-in-recent-decades/.

Pew Research Center. "The Social Life of Health Information, 2011," May 12, 2011. https://www.pewresearch.org/internet/2011/05/12/the-social-life-of-health-information-2011/.

Potts, Malcolm. "Birth Control | Description, History, Types, & Effectiveness," *Encyclopedia Britannica*, July 11, 2024. https://www.britannica.com/science/birth-control/Ethics-and-the-influence-of-religious-systems.

Power to Decide. "Impacts of the Domestic Gag Rule," n.d. https://powertodecide.org/sites/default/files/2020-10/Impacts%20of%20the%20Domestic%20Gag%20Rule_Factsheet.pdf.

Prestin, Abby, Sana N. Vieux, and Wen-Ying Sylvia Chou. "Is Online Health Activity Alive and Well or Flatlining? Findings From 10 Years of the Health Information National Trends Survey," *Journal of Health Communication* 20, no. 7 (June 4, 2015): 790–8. https://doi.org/10.1080/10810730.2015.1018590.

"Recommendations for Group-Based Behavioral Interventions to Prevent Adolescent Pregnancy, Human Immunodeficiency Virus, and Other Sexually

Transmitted Infections," *American Journal of Preventive Medicine* 42, no. 3 (March 1, 2012): 304–7. https://doi.org/10.1016/j.amepre.2011.11.003.

Ronald Reagan Presidential Library & Museum. "Facts About Ronald Reagan," n.d. https://www.reaganlibrary.gov/reagans/ronald-reagan/facts-about-ronald-reagan.

Rosoff, J. I. "The Politics of Birth Control," *Family Planning Perspectives* 20, no. 6 (1990): 312–97. https://pubmed.ncbi.nlm.nih.gov/3068073/.

Secura, Gina M., Tiffany Adams, Christina M. Buckel, Qiuhong Zhao, and Jeffrey F. Peipert. "Change in Sexual Behavior With Provision of No-Cost Contraception," *Obstetrics and Gynecology* 123, no. 4 (April 1, 2014): 771–6. https://doi.org/10.1097/aog.0000000000000184.

Stanger-Hall, Kathrin F., and David W. Hall. "Abstinence-Only Education and Teen Pregnancy Rates: Why We Need Comprehensive Sex Education in the U.S.," *PLoS ONE* 6, no. 10 (October 14, 2011): e24658. https://doi.org/10.1371/journal.pone.0024658.

"Statement on Signing the Family Planning Services and Population Research Act of 1970. | The American Presidency Project," December 26, 1970. https://www.presidency.ucsb.edu/documents/statement-signing-the-family-planning-services-and-population-research-act-1970.

Waxman, Olivia B. "This Peanuts Strip Offers a Window Into Ronald Reagan's Changing Views on Abortion," *TIME*, June 1, 2021. https://time.com/6047987/peanuts-history-reagan-abortion/.

Chapter 4

Alptraum, Lux. "Why It's So Hard to Invent a New Kind of Condom (in the US, Anyway)," *Vice*, June 16, 2016. https://www.vice.com/en/article/vv73ex/new-kind-of-condom-in-the-us-anyway-lelo-hex-charlie-sheen.

Barber, Regina G. "In The Hunt for a Male Contraceptive, Scientists Look to Stop Sperm in Their Tracks," *NPR*, December 4, 2022. https://www.npr.org/sections/health-shots/2022/12/04/1140512789/birth-control-male-contraceptive-sperm.

Byrne, K. "Medical Records in Litigation: The Dalkon Shield Story," *PubMed*, February 1, 1992, https://pubmed.ncbi.nlm.nih.gov/10117045/.

Center for Male Contraceptive Research & Development. "FAQs on Hormonal Male Contraception," https://www.malecontraception.center/faqs.

ClinicalTrials.gov. "Study of Daily Application of Nestorone® (NES) and Testosterone (T) Combination Gel for Male Contraception," September 8, 2023. https://clinicaltrials.gov/study/NCT03452111.

Dittrick Medical History Center. "19th Century Artifacts," *College of Arts and Science*, n.d. https://artsci.case.edu/dittrick/online-exhibits/history-of-birth-control/contraception-in-america-1800-1900/19th-century-artifacts/.

Dittrick Medical History Center. "Condoms and Sponges," *College of Arts and Sciences*, n.d. https://artsci.case.edu/dittrick/online-exhibits/history-of-birth-control/contraception-in-america-1900-1950/condoms-and-sponges/.

Eisenberg, Michael L., Jillian T. Henderson, John K. Amory, James F. Smith, and Thomas J. Walsh. "Racial Differences in Vasectomy Utilization in the United States: Data From the National Survey of Family Growth," *Urology* 74, no. 5 (November 1, 2009): 1020–4. https://doi.org/10.1016/j.urology.2009.06.042.

Eunice Kennedy Shriver National Institute of Child Health and Human Development. "Spotlight: One Year and Counting: Male Birth Control Study Reaches Milestone," *US Department of Health and Human Services*, August 2, 2022. https://www.nichd.nih.gov/newsroom/news/080222-NEST.

Glasier, A. F., R. Anakwe, D. Everington, C. W. Martin, Z. Van Der Spuy, L. Cheng, P. C. Ho, and R. A. Anderson. "Would Women Trust Their Partners to Use a Male Pill?" *Human Reproduction* 15, no. 3 (March 1, 2000): 646–9. https://doi.org/10.1093/humrep/15.3.646.

Gorvett, Zaria. "The Weird Reasons There Still Isn't a Male Contraceptive Pill," *BBC*, February 16, 2023. https://www.bbc.com/future/article/20230216-the-weird-reasons-male-birth-control-pills-are-scorned.

Guttmacher Institute. "Contraceptive Effectiveness in the United States," August 24, 2022. https://www.guttmacher.org/fact-sheet/contraceptive-effectiveness-united-states.

Haddad, Lisa B., John W. Townsend, and Regine Sitruk-Ware. "Contraceptive Technologies: Looking Ahead to New Approaches to Increase Options for Family Planning," *Clinical Obstetrics & Gynecology* 64, no. 3 (May 11, 2021): 435–48. https://doi.org/10.1097/grf.0000000000000628.

Huang, Pien. "A New, Experimental Approach to Male Birth Control Immobilizes Sperm," *NPR*, February 18, 2023. https://www.npr.org/sections/health-shots/2023/02/17/1157841943/researchers-found-a-new-approach-to-a-male-contraceptive-used-only-by-mice-so-fa.

Khan, Fahd, Saheel Mukhtar, Ian K. Dickinson, and Seshadri Sriprasad. "The Story of the Condom," *Indian Journal of Urology* 29, no. 1 (January 1, 2013): 12. https://doi.org/10.4103/0970-1591.109976.

Khilwani, Barkha, Ayesha Badar, Abdul S. Ansari, and Nirmal K. Lohiya. "RISUG® as a Male Contraceptive: Journey From Bench to Bedside," *Basic and Clinical Andrology* 30, no. 1 (February 13, 2020): 2. https://doi.org/10.1186/s12610-020-0099-1.

Krismann, Carol H. "Dalkon Shield | Contraceptive Device & Health Risks," *Encyclopedia Britannica*, December 4, 2013. https://www.britannica.com/science/Dalkon-Shield.

Lieberman, Hallie, "A Short History of the Condom," *JSTOR Daily*, June 21, 2018. https://daily.jstor.org/short-history-of-the-condom/.

"Male Contraceptive Implanted at Epworth Freemasons in World First," *EPWorth*, November 10, 2022. https://www.epworth.org.au/newsroom/male-contraceptive-implanted-at-epworth-freemasons-in-world-first.

Male Contraceptive Initiative. "Contraline," n.d. https://www.malecontraceptive.org/contraline.html.

Male Contraceptive Initiative. "Drug Development Pipeline," n.d. https://www.malecontraceptive.org/the-drug-development-pipeline.html.

Male Contraceptive Initiative, "Interest Among U.S. Men for New Male Contraceptive Options Consumer Research Study," February 2019. https://www.malecontraceptive.org/uploads/1/3/1/9/131958006/mci_consumerresearchstudy.pdf.

Male Contraceptive Initiative. "Male Contraceptive Initiative Invests $1 Million in Contraline to Conduct Clinical Trial for Long-Lasting, Non-Hormonal Male Contraceptive," November 18, 2020. https://www.malecontraceptive.org/press-releases/male-contraceptive-initiative-invests-1-million-in-contraline-to-conduct-clinical-trial-for-long-lasting-non-hormonal-male-contraceptive.

Male Contraceptive Initiative. "Non-Hormonal, Reversible Male Contraception Database," n.d. https://www.malecontraceptive.org/nhrmc-database.html.

PBS. "The Puerto Rico Pill Trials," *American Experience* | PBS, March 13, 2018. https://www.pbs.org/wgbh/americanexperience/features/pill-puerto-rico-pill-trials/.

Pisac, Anna, and Natalia Wilson. "FDA Device Oversight From 1906 to the Present," *The AMA Journal of Ethic* 23, no. 9 (September 1, 2021): E712–20. https://doi.org/10.1001/amajethics.2021.712.

Potts, Malcolm. "Birth Control | Description, History, Types, & Effectiveness," *Encyclopedia Britannica*, July 11, 2024. https://www.britannica.com/science/birth-control/Ethics-and-the-influence-of-religious-systems.

Reynolds-Wright, John J., Nicholas J. Cameron, and Richard A. Anderson. "Will Men Use Novel Male Contraceptive Methods and Will Women Trust Them? A Systematic Review," *The Journal of Sex Research* 58, no. 7 (April 26, 2021): 838–49. https://doi.org/10.1080/00224499.2021.1905764.

Service, C. Austin, Dhruv Puri, Tung-Chin Hsieh, and Darshan P. Patel. "Emerging Concepts in Male Contraception: A Narrative Review of Novel, Hormonal and Non-hormonal Options," *Therapeutic Advances in*

Reproductive Health 17 (January 1, 2023): 263349412211383. https://doi.org/10.1177/26334941221138323.

U.S. Food and Drug Administration. "Birth Control Guide (Chart)," *FDA*, May 2024. http://www.fda.gov/birthcontrol.

Wang, Christina, Mario P. R. Festin, and Ronald S. Swerdloff. "Male Hormonal Contraception: Where Are We Now?" *Current Obstetrics and Gynecology Reports* 5, no. 1 (January 29, 2016): 38–47. https://doi.org/10.1007/s13669-016-0140-8.

World Medical Association. "WMA – the World Medical Association-WMA Declaration of Helsinki – Ethical Principles for Medical Research Involving Human Subjects," *WMA*, June 1964. https://www.wma.net/policies-post/wma-declaration-of-helsinki-ethical-principles-for-medical-research-involving-human-subjects/.

Wouters, Olivier J., Martin McKee, and Jeroen Luyten. "Estimated Research and Development Investment Needed to Bring a New Medicine to Market, 2009–2018," *JAMA* 323, no. 9 (March 3, 2020): 844. https://doi.org/10.1001/jama.2020.1166.

Zhang, Xinyuan, and Michael L. Eisenberg. "Vasectomy Utilization in Men Aged 18–45 Declined Between 2002 and 2017: Results From the United States National Survey for Family Growth Data," *Andrology* 10, no. 1 (August 31, 2021): 137–42. https://doi.org/10.1111/andr.13093.

Chapter 5

ACOG. "Combined Hormonal Birth Control: Pill, Patch, and Ring," n.d. https://www.acog.org/womens-health/faqs/combined-hormonal-birth-control-pill-patch-ring.

Bailey, Martha J. "Fifty Years of Family Planning: New Evidence on the Long-Run Effects of Increasing Access to Contraception," *Brookings Papers on Economic Activity* 2013, no. 1 (March 1, 2013): 341–409. https://doi.org/10.1353/eca.2013.0001.

Blakemore, Erin, and Erin Blakemore. "The First Birth Control Pill Used Puerto Rican Women as Guinea Pigs," *HISTORY*, August 24, 2023. https://www.history.com/news/birth-control-pill-history-puerto-rico-enovid.

Centers for Disease Control and Prevention. "Margaret Sanger," *MMWR*, December 3, 1999. https://www.cdc.gov/mmwr/preview/mmwrhtml/mm4847bx.htm.

Cooper, Danielle B., and Preeti Patel. "Oral Contraceptive Pills," *StatPearls - NCBI Bookshelf*, February 29, 2024. https://www.ncbi.nlm.nih.gov/books/NBK430882/.

Daniels, Kimberly, William Mosher, and Jo Jones. "Contraceptive Methods Women Have Ever Used: United States, 1982–2010," *National Health Statistics Reports* 62, February 14, 2023. https://www.cdc.gov/nchs/data/nhsr/nhsr062.pdf.

Dittrick Medical History Center. "Cervical Caps and Diaphragms," n.d. https://artsci.case.edu/dittrick/online-exhibits/history-of-birth-control/contraception-in-america-1900-1950/cervical-caps-and-diaphragms/.

Encyclopaedia Britannica. "Margaret Sanger | Biography, Birth Control, & Significance," *Encyclopedia Britannica*, July 4, 2024. https://www.britannica.com/biography/Margaret-Sanger.

Guttmacher Institute. "Guttmacher Releases Latest Findings From the Reproductive Health Impact Study Documenting the Effects of the Domestic Gag Rule and Other Restrictions on Family Planning Providers," September 1, 2022. https://www.guttmacher.org/news-release/2022/guttmacher-releases-latest-findings-reproductive-health-impact-study-documenting.

HHS Office of Population Affairs. "Title X Family Planning Annual Report 2022 National Summary," October 2023. https://opa.hhs.gov/sites/default/files/2023-10/2022-FPAR-National-Summary.pdf.

HHS Office of Population Affairs. "Title X Service Grants," n.d. https://opa.hhs.gov/grant-programs/title-x-service-grants.

HHS Office of Population Affairs. "Title X Turns 50," n.d. https://opa.hhs.gov/grant-programs/title-x-service-grants/title-x-turns-50.

Junod, Suzanne White. "FDA's Approval of the First Oral Contraceptive, Enovid," *U.S Food and Drug Administration*, 1998. https://www.fda.gov/media/110456/download.

Katz, Esther. "Sanger, Margaret (1879–1966), Birth Control Advocate," *American National Biography*, February 2000. https://doi.org/10.1093/anb/9780198606697.article.1500598.

Kelly, Mary Louise, and Mary Ziegler. "The History of Title X Throughout U.S. History," *All Things Considered* | NPR, May 18, 2018. https://www.npr.org/2018/05/18/612441155/the-history-of-title-x-throughout-u-s-history.

Knowles, Jon, et al. "A History of Birth Control Methods," *Planned Parenthood Federation of America*, 2012. https://www.plannedparenthood.org/files/2613/9611/6275/History_of_BC_Methods.pdf.

Michals, Debra. "Biography: Margaret Sanger," *National Women's History Museum*, 2017 https://www.womenshistory.org/education-resources/biographies/margaret-sanger.

PBS. "A Timeline of Contraception," *American Experience* | PBS, March 13, 2018. https://www.pbs.org/wgbh/americanexperience/features/pill-timeline/.

PBS. "Dr. John Rock (1890–1984)," *American Experience* | PBS, March 13, 2018. https://www.pbs.org/wgbh/americanexperience/features/pill-dr-john-rock-1890-1984/.

PBS. "Eugenics and Birth Control," *American Experience* | PBS, March 13, 2018. https://www.pbs.org/wgbh/americanexperience/features/pill-eugenics-and-birth-control/.

PBS. "The FDA Approves the Pill," *American Experience* | PBS, March 13, 2018. https://www.pbs.org/wgbh/americanexperience/features/pill-us-food-and-drug-administration-approves-pill/.

PBS. "Gregory Pincus (1903–1967)," *American Experience* | PBS, March 13, 2018. https://www.pbs.org/wgbh/americanexperience/features/gregory-pincus-1903-1967/.

PBS. "Katharine Dexter McCormick (1875–1967)," *American Experience* | PBS, March 13, 2018. https://www.pbs.org/wgbh/americanexperience/features/pill-katharine-dexter-mccormick-1875-1967/.

PBS. "Margaret Sanger (1879–1966)," *American Experience* | PBS, March 13, 2018. https://www.pbs.org/wgbh/americanexperience/features/pill-margaret-sanger-1879-1966/.

PBS. "The Pill and the Sexual Revolution," *American Experience* | PBS, March 13, 2018. https://www.pbs.org/wgbh/americanexperience/features/pill-and-sexual-revolution/.

PBS. "The Pill in America," *American Experience* | *PBS,* March 13, 2018. https://www.pbs.org/wgbh/americanexperience/features/pill-america/.

PBS. "The Puerto Rico Pill Trials," *American Experience* | PBS, March 13, 2018. https://www.pbs.org/wgbh/americanexperience/features/pill-puerto-rico-pill-trials/.

PBS. "Roots of the Pill," *American Experience* | PBS, March 13, 2018. https://www.pbs.org/wgbh/americanexperience/features/roots-pill/.

Planned Parenthood. "The Birth Control Pill: A History," 2015. https://www.plannedparenthood.org/files/1514/3518/7100/Pill_History_FactSheet.pdf.

United Nations Department of Economic and Social Affairs. "Contraceptive Use by Method 2019 Data Booklet," *UN*, 2019. https://www.un.org/development/desa/pd/sites/www.un.org.development.desa.pd/files/files/documents/2020/Jan/un_2019_contraceptiveusebymethod_databooklet.pdf.

U.S. Food and Drug Administration. "FDA Approves First Nonprescription Daily Oral Contraceptive," *FDA*, July 13, 2023. https://www.fda.gov/news-events/press-announcements/fda-approves-first-nonprescription-daily-oral-contraceptive.

U.S. Food and Drug Administration. "FDA Policy for the Protection of Human Subjects," *FDA*, June 18, 1991. https://www.fda.gov/science-research/clinical-trials-and-human-subject-protection/fda-policy-protection-human-subjects.

Vamos, Cheryl A., Ellen M. Daley, Kay M. Perrin, Charles S. Mahan, and Eric R. Buhi. "Approaching 4 Decades of Legislation in the National Family Planning Program: An Analysis of Title X's History From 1970 to 2008," *American Journal of Public Health* 101, no. 11 (November 1, 2011): 2027–37. https://doi.org/10.2105/ajph.2011.300202.

Yanagimachi, Ryuzo. "M.C. Chang: A Pioneer of Mammalian in Vitro Fertilization," *Molecular Reproduction and Development* 83, no. 10 (October 1, 2016): 846–9. https://doi.org/10.1002/mrd.22749.

Chapter 6

American Public Health Association. "Opposing Coercion in Contraceptive Access and Care to Promote Reproductive Health Equity," *Policy Number 202110*, October 26, 2021. https://apha.org/policies-and-advocacy/public-health-policy-statements/policy-database/2022/01/07/opposing-coercion-in-contraceptive-access-and-care-to-promote-reproductive-health-equity.

Barot, Sneha. "Governmental Coercion in Reproductive Decision Making: See It Both Ways," *Guttmacher Policy Review* 15, no. 4 (August 18, 2023). https://www.guttmacher.org/gpr/2012/10/governmental-coercion-reproductive-decision-making-see-it-both-ways.

Birthright, Inc. "Birthright, Inc. | University of Minnesota Archival Collections Guides," n.d. https://archives.lib.umn.edu/agents/corporate_entities/3413.

Borrero, Sonya, Nikki Zite, and Mitchell D. Creinin. "Federally Funded Sterilization: Time to Rethink Policy?" *American Journal of Public Health* 102, no. 10 (October 1, 2012): 1822–5. https://doi.org/10.2105/ajph.2012.300850.

Center for the History of Medicine (Francis A. Countway Library of Medicine). "Clarence James Gamble Papers," *Harvard University Library*, n.d. https://hollisarchives.lib.harvard.edu/repositories/14/resources/9255.

Dehlendorf, Christine, Aletha Y. Akers, Sonya Borrero, Lisa S. Callegari, Denicia Cadena, Anu Manchikanti Gomez, Jamie Hart, et al. "Evolving the Preconception Health Framework," *Obstetrics and Gynecology* 137, no. 2 (January 5, 2021): 234–9. https://doi.org/10.1097/aog.0000000000004255.

Early, Rosalind. "The Sweat and Blood of Fannie Lou Hamer," *Humanities, The Magazine of the National Endowment for the Humanities* 42, no. 1 (Winter 2021).

Fair, Alexander. "The Sterilization of Carrie Buck," *Origins: Current Events in Historical Perspective, The Ohio State University*, 2022. https://origins.osu.edu/read/sterilization-carrie-buck?language_content_entity=en.

Gillespie, Katherine. "Defining Reproductive Freedom for Women 'Living Under a Microscope': Relf V. Weinberger and the Involuntary Sterilization of Poor Women of Color," *University of Georgetown*, 2000. https://repository.library.georgetown.edu/handle/10822/1051142.

Gold, Rachel Benson. "Guarding Against Coercion While Ensuring Access: A Delicate Balance," *Guttmacher Policy Review* 17, no. 3 (September 2, 2014): 8–14. https://www.guttmacher.org/gpr/2014/09/guarding-against-coercion-while-ensuring-access-delicate-balance.

Justia Law. "Buck V. Bell, 274 U.S. 200 (1927)," n.d. https://supreme.justia.com/cases/federal/us/274/200/.

Karasic, Dan. "Legal and Identity Documents," *University of California, San Francisco*, June 17, 2016. https://transcare.ucsf.edu/guidelines/legal.

Movement Advancement Project. "Equality Maps: Identity Document Laws and Policies," *Movement Advancement Project*, n.d. https://www.mapresearch.org/equality-maps/identity_document_laws.

Narea, Nicole. "The Outcry Over ICE and Hysterectomies, Explained," *Vox*, September 18, 2020. https://www.vox.com/policy-and-politics/2020/9/15/21437805/whistleblower-hysterectomies-nurse-irwin-ice.

National Human Genome Research Institute. "Eugenics and Scientific Racism," *National Human Genome Research Institutem*, n.d. https://www.genome.gov/about-genomics/fact-sheets/Eugenics-and-Scientific-Racism.

National Partnership for Women and Families. "Past as Present: America's Sordid History of Medical Reproductive Abuse and Experimentation," *National Partnership for Women and Families*, September 2020. https://nationalpartnership.org/wp-content/uploads/2023/02/past-as-present-americas-sordid-history-of-medical-reproductive-abuse-and-experimentation.pdf.

National Public Radio. "The Supreme Court Ruling That Led to 70,000 Forced Sterilizations," *Fresh Air | NPR*, March 7, 2016. https://www.npr.org/sections/health-shots/2016/03/07/469478098/the-supreme-court-ruling-that-led-to-70-000-forced-sterilizations.

New York Times. "3 Carolina Doctors Are Under Inquiry In Sterilization of Welfare Mothers," July 22, 1973. https://www.nytimes.com/1973/07/22/archives/3-carolina-doctors-are-under-inquiry-in-sterilization-of-welfare.html.

New York Times. "Sterilization of Black Mother of 3 Stirs Aiken, S.C.," August 1, 1973. https://www.nytimes.com/1973/08/01/archives/sterilization-of-black-mother-of-3-stirs-aiken-sc-residents-angered.html.

PBS. "Finding Carrie Buck," *American Experience | PBS*, November 2, 2018. https://www.pbs.org/wgbh/americanexperience/features/eugenics-finding-carrie-buck/.

Raine, Susan P. "Federal Sterilization Policy: Unintended Consequences," The *AMA Journal of Ethic* 14, no. 2 (February 1, 2012): 152–7. https://doi.org/10.1001/virtualmentor.2012.14.2.mhst1-1202.

Reilly, Philip R. "Eugenics and Involuntary Sterilization: 1907–2015," *Annual Review of Genomics and Human Genetics* 16, no. 1 (August 24, 2015): 351–68. https://doi.org/10.1146/annurev-genom-090314-024930.

SisterSong. "About Us — SisterSong," n.d. https://www.sistersong.net/about-x2.

Stern, Alexandra Minna. "STERILIZED in the Name of Public Health," *American Journal of Public Health* 95, no. 7 (July 1, 2005): 1128–38. https://doi.org/10.2105/ajph.2004.041608.

Southern Poverty Law Center. "Relf V. Weinberger," n.d. https://www.splcenter.org/seeking-justice/case-docket/relf-v-weinberger.

University of North Carolina. "Collection Title: Human Betterment League of North Carolina, Inc. Records, 1947–1988," *Wilson Special Collections Library*, n.d. https://finding-aids.lib.unc.edu/04519/.

University of Virginia. "Carrie Buck Revisited and Virginia's Expression of Regret for Eugenics," *HIstorical Collections at the Claude Moore Health Sciences Library*, 2004. https://exhibits.hsl.virginia.edu/eugenics/5-epilogue/.

Chapter 7

Ahmed, Saifuddin, and Özge Tunçalp. "Burden of Obstetric Fistula: From Measurement to Action," *The Lancet Global Health* 3, no. 5 (May 1, 2015): e243–4. https://doi.org/10.1016/s2214-109x(15)70105-1.

American Civil Liberties Union. "Norplant: A New Contraceptive With the Potential for Abuse," January 31, 1994. https://wp.api.aclu.org/documents/norplant-new-contraceptive-potential-abuse.

American Public Health Association. "Opposing Coercion in Contraceptive Access and Care to Promote Reproductive Health Equity," *Policy Number 202110*, October 26, 2021 https://apha.org/policies-and-advocacy/public-health-policy-statements/policy-database/2022/01/07/opposing-coercion-in-contraceptive-access-and-care-to-promote-reproductive-health-equity.

References

Brandi, Kristyn, and Liza Fuentes. "The History of Tiered-effectiveness Contraceptive Counseling and the Importance of Patient-centered Family Planning Care," *American Journal of Obstetrics and Gynecology* 222, no. 4 (April 1, 2020): S873–7. https://doi.org/10.1016/j.ajog.2019.11.1271.

Cappello, Olivia. "Powerful Contraception, Complicated Programs: Preventing Coercive Promotion of Long-Acting Reversible Contraceptives," *Guttmacher Policy Review*, May 10, 2021. https://www.guttmacher.org/gpr/2021/05/powerful-contraception-complicated-programs-preventing-coercive-promotion-long-acting.

The College of Physicians of Philadelphia. "James Marion Sims: Father of Modern Gynecology or Abuser?" n.d. https://collegeofphysicians.org/programs/education-blog/james-marion-sims-father-modern-gynecology-or-abuser.

Corbett, Megan. "A History: The IUD," *Reproductive Health Access Project Blog*, January 2013, Updated March 2024. https://www.reproductiveaccess.org/2024/03/a-history-the-iud/.

Dehlendorf, Christine, Rachel Ruskin, Kevin Grumbach, Eric Vittinghoff, Kirsten Bibbins-Domingo, Dean Schillinger, and Jody Steinauer. "Recommendations for Intrauterine Contraception: A Randomized Trial of the Effects of Patients' Race/Ethnicity and Socioeconomic Status," *American Journal of Obstetrics and Gynecology* 203, no. 4 (October 1, 2010): 319. e1–319.e8. https://doi.org/10.1016/j.ajog.2010.05.009.

Domonoske, Camila. "'Father of Gynecology,' Who Experimented on Slaves, No Longer on Pedestal in NYC," *NPR*, April 17, 2018. https://www.npr.org/sections/thetwo-way/2018/04/17/603163394/-father-of-gynecology-who-experimented-on-slaves-no-longer-on-pedestal-in-nyc.

Eeckhaut, Mieke C. W., and Yuko Hara. "Reproductive Oppression Enters the Twenty-First Century: Pressure to Use Long-Acting Reversible Contraception (LARC) in the Context of 'LARC First,'" *Socius* 9 (January 1, 2023). https://doi.org/10.1177/23780231231180378.

Eeckhaut, Mieke C. W., Michael S. Rendall, and Polina Zvavitch. "Women's Use of Long-Acting Reversible Contraception for Birth Timing and Birth Stopping," *Demography* 58, no. 4 (July 12, 2021): 1327–46. https://doi.org/10.1215/00703370-9386084.

Gold, Rachel Benson. "Guarding Against Coercion While Ensuring Access: A Delicate Balance," *Guttmacher Policy Review* 17, no. 3 (September 2, 2014). https://www.guttmacher.org/gpr/2014/09/guarding-against-coercion-while-ensuring-access-delicate-balance.

Guttmacher Institute. "FDA Gives Final Approval to Depo Amid Concerns Over Safety, Cost and Coercion," *Guttmacher Institute* 12, no. 17 (1992): 2–3.

Higgins, Jenny A., Renee D. Kramer, and Kristin M. Ryder. "Provider Bias in Long-Acting Reversible Contraception (LARC) Promotion and Removal: Perceptions of Young Adult Women," *American Journal of Public Health* 106, no. 11 (November 1, 2016): 1932–7. https://doi.org/10.2105/ajph.2016.303393.

Hoffman, Kelly M., Sophie Trawalter, Jordan R. Axt, and M. Norman Oliver. "Racial Bias in Pain Assessment and Treatment Recommendations, and False Beliefs About Biological Differences Between Blacks and Whites," *Proceedings of the National Academy of Sciences of the United States of America* 113, no. 16 (April 4, 2016): 4296–301. https://doi.org/10.1073/pnas.1516047113.

Holland, Brynn. "The 'Father of Modern Gynecology' Performed Shocking Experiments on Enslaved Women," *HISTORY*, August 29, 2017. https://www.history.com/news/the-father-of-modern-gynecology-performed-shocking-experiments-on-slaves.

Nduka, Ifunanya Roseline, Nasreen Ali, Isabella Kabasinguzi, and David Abdy. "The Psycho-social Impact of Obstetric Fistula and Available Support for Women Residing in Nigeria: A Systematic Review," *BMC Women's Health* 23, no. 1 (February 25, 2023). https://doi.org/10.1186/s12905-023-02220-7.

New-York Historical Society. "Life Story: Anarcha, Betsy, and Lucy," *NY History*, n.d. https://wams.nyhistory.org/a-nation-divided/antebellum/anarcha-betsy-lucy/.

Kaiser Family Foundation. "DMPA Contraceptive Injection: Use and Coverage," *KFF*, May 30, 2024. https://www.kff.org/womens-health-policy/fact-sheet/dmpa-contraceptive-injection-use-and-coverage/.

Roberts, Dorothy. *Killing the Black Body*. Vintage. December, 1998.

Scully, Judith A. M. "Black Women and the Development of International Reproductive Health Norms," in *Black Women and International Law: Deliberate Interactions, Movements and Actions*, edited by J. I. Levitt, 225–49. Cambridge: Cambridge University Press, 2015. https://doi.org/10.1017/cbo9781139108751.013.

SisterSong. "Justice Statement," n.d. https://www.sistersong.net/justice-statement.

SisterSong. "Reproductive Justice," n.d. https://www.sistersong.net/reproductive-justice.

"SisterSong and National Women's Health Network. Long-Acting Reversible Contraception Statement of Principles," n.d. https://nwhn.org/wp-content/uploads/2024/01/LARC-Statement-of-Principles.pdf.

Skloot, Rebecca. *The Immortal Life of Henrietta Lacks*. Crown, March, 2011.

Sonfield, Adam. "Popularity Disparity: Attitudes About the IUD in Europe and the United States," *Guttmacher Policy Review* 10, no. 4 (November 8, 2007): 19–24.

Spain, Janine E., Jeffrey F. Peipert, Tessa Madden, Jenifer E. Allsworth, and Gina M. Secura. "The Contraceptive CHOICE Project: Recruiting Women at Highest Risk for Unintended Pregnancy and Sexually Transmitted Infection," *Journal of Womens Health* 19, no. 12 (December 1, 2010): 2233–8. https://doi.org/10.1089/jwh.2010.2146.

Urell, Aaryn. "Tuskegee Syphilis Experiment," *Equal Justice Initiative*, October 31, 2020. https://eji.org/news/history-racial-injustice-tuskegee-syphilis-experiment/.

Wall, L L. "The Medical Ethics of Dr J Marion Sims: A Fresh Look at the Historical Record," *Journal of Medical Ethics* 32, no. 6 (May 26, 2006): 346–50. https://doi.org/10.1136/jme.2005.012559.

Wingert, Pat. "The Norplant Debate," *Newsweek*, February 14, 1993. https://www.newsweek.com/norplant-debate-195258.

World Health Organization: WHO. "Obstetric Fistula," February 19, 2018. https://www.who.int/news-room/facts-in-pictures/detail/10-facts-on-obstetric-fistula.

Zellars, Rachel. "Black Subjectivity and the Origins of American Gynecology," *AAIHS - African American Intellectual History Society*, May 31, 2018. https://www.aaihs.org/black-subjectivity-and-the-origins-of-american-gynecology/.

Chapter 8

Advocates for Youth. "New Data: Most Young People Face Barriers to Birth Control Access," *Advocates for Youth*, September 26, 2022. https://www.advocatesforyouth.org/press-releases/most-young-people-face-barriers-to-birth-control-access/.

Ahmed, Zara. "The Unprecedented Expansion of the Global Gag Rule: Trampling Rights, Health and Free Speech," *Guttmacher Policy Review*, 23. April 28, 2020. https://www.guttmacher.org/gpr/2020/04/unprecedented-expansion-global-gag-rule-trampling-rights-health-and-free-speech.

American College of Obstetricians and Gynecologists. "Access to Contraception," *Committee on Health Care for Underserved Women*, 2015 (reaffirmed 2022). https://www.acog.org/clinical/clinical-guidance/committee-opinion/articles/2015/01/access-to-contraception.

American College of Obstetricians and Gynecologists. "Reproductive and Sexual Coercion," *Committee on Health Care for Underserved Women*, 2013 (reaffirmed 2022). https://www.acog.org/clinical/clinical-guidance/committee-opinion/articles/2013/02/reproductive-and-sexual-coercion.

American Public Health Association. "Opposing Coercion in Contraceptive Access and Care to Promote Reproductive Health Equity," *Policy Number 202110*, October 26, 2021. https://apha.org/policies-and-advocacy/public-health-policy-statements/policy-database/2022/01/07/opposing-coercion-in-contraceptive-access-and-care-to-promote-reproductive-health-equity.

Barot, Sneha. "Governmental Coercion in Reproductive Decision Making: See It Both Ways," *Guttmacher Policy Review* 15, no. 4: (August 18, 2023): 7–12. https://www.guttmacher.org/gpr/2012/10/governmental-coercion-reproductive-decision-making-see-it-both-ways.

Basile, Kathleen C., Sharon G. Smith, Yang Liu, Elizabeth Miller, and Marcie-Jo Kresnow. "Prevalence of Intimate Partner Reproductive Coercion in the United States: Racial and Ethnic Differences," *Journal of Interpersonal Violence* 36, no. 21–22 (December 6, 2019): NP12324–41. https://doi.org/10.1177/0886260519888205.

Centers for Disease Control and Prevention. "Unintended Pregnancy," May 15, 2024. https://www.cdc.gov/reproductive-health/hcp/unintended-pregnancy/index.html.

Curtis, K. M., Nguyen, A. T., Tepper, N. K., et al. "U.S. Selected Practice Recommendations for Contraceptive Use, 2024," *MMWR Recomm Rep* 73, no. 3 (2024): 1–77. http://dx.doi.org/10.15585/mmwr.rr7303a1.

Diep, Karen, Michelle Long, and Alina Salganicoff. "Oral Contraceptive Pills: Access and Availability," *KFF*, March 20, 2024. https://www.kff.org/womens-health-policy/issue-brief/oral-contraceptive-pills-access-and-availability/.

Felix, Mabel Laurie Sobel, and Alina Salganicoff. "The Right to Contraception: State and Federal Actions, Misinformation, and the Courts," *KFF*, May 28, 2024. https://www.kff.org/womens-health-policy/issue-brief/the-right-to-contraception-state-and-federal-actions-misinformation-and-the-courts/.

Frederiksen, Brittni, Usha Ranji, Michelle Long, Karen Diep, and Alina Salganicoff. "Contraception in the United States: A Closer Look at Experiences, Preferences, and Coverage," *KFF*, November 18, 2022. https://www.kff.org/womens-health-policy/report/contraception-in-the-united-states-a-closer-look-at-experiences-preferences-and-coverage/.

Guttmacher Institute. "An Overview of Consent to Reproductive Health Services by Young People," *Guttmacher Institute*, August 30, 2023. https://www.guttmacher.org/state-policy/explore/overview-minors-consent-law.

Guttmacher Institute. "Cost Continues to Pose Significant Barriers to Contraceptive Access," *Guttmacher Institute*, May 24, 2023. https://www.guttmacher.org/news-release/2023/cost-continues-pose-significant-barriers-contraceptive-access.

Guttmacher Institute. "Minors' Access to Contraceptive Services," *Guttmacher Institute*, August 30, 2023. https://www.guttmacher.org/state-policy/explore/minors-access-contraceptive-services.

Guttmacher Institute. "Pharmacist-Prescribed Contraceptives," *Guttmacher Institute*, August 31, 2023. https://www.guttmacher.org/state-policy/explore/pharmacist-prescribed-contraceptives.

Guttmacher Institute. "State Family Planning Funding Restrictions," *Guttmacher Institute*, September 1, 2023. https://www.guttmacher.org/state-policy/explore/state-family-planning-funding-restrictions.

HHS Office of Population Affairs. "Title X Program Funding History," *HHS*, n.d. https://opa.hhs.gov/grant-programs/archive/title-x-program-archive/title-x-program-funding-history.

HHS Office of Population Affairs. "Title X Service Grants," *HHS*, n.d. https://opa.hhs.gov/grant-programs/title-x-service-grants.

Human Rights Watch. "Iran: Population Law Violates Women's Rights," *HRW*, November 10, 2021. https://www.hrw.org/news/2021/11/10/iran-population-law-violates-womens-rights.

Kavanaugh, Megan L., and Amy Friedrich-Karnik. "Has the Fall of Roe Changed Contraceptive Access and Use? New Research From Four US States Offers Critical Insights," *Health Affairs Scholar*, February 8, 2024. https://doi.org/10.1093/haschl/qxae016.

National Conference of State Legislatures. "State Contraception Policies," *NCSL*, September 7, 2023. https://www.ncsl.org/health/state-contraception-policies.

National Women's Law Center. "Policy Brief: Remove Barriers and Expand Access to Birth Control," *NWLC*, 2021. https://nwlc.org/wp-content/uploads/2021/01/BirthControl_FS_nwlc_LegislativePacketEW1.pdf

PerryUndem Research/Communication. "Views on Birth Control Report," *PerryUndem*, n.d. https://view.publitas.com/perryundem-research-communication/views-on-birth-control-report-pdf/page/1.

Planned Parenthood Action Fund. "Stories: The Benefits of Birth Control," *Planned Parenthood*, n.d. https://www.plannedparenthoodaction.org/issues/birth-control/birth-control-stories

Santelli, John et al., "Abstinence-Only-Until-Marriage Policies and Programs: An Updated Position Paper of the Society for Adolescent Health and Medicine," *Journal of Adolescent Health* 61, no. 3 (September 1, 2017): 400–3. https://doi.org/10.1016/j.jadohealth.2017.06.001.

Swan, Laura E. T., Annelise Mennicke, and Youngmi Kim. "Reproductive Coercion and Interpersonal Violence Victimization Experiences Among College Students," *Journal of Interpersonal Violence* 36, no. 23–4 (January 10, 2020): 11281–303. https://doi.org/10.1177/0886260519898424.

Willie, Tiara C., Kamila A. Alexander, Amy Caplon, Trace S. Kershaw, Cara B. Safon, Rachel W. Galvao, Clair Kaplan, Abigail Caldwell, and Sarah K. Calabrese. "Birth Control Sabotage as a Correlate of Women's Sexual Health Risk: An Exploratory Study," *Women's Health Issues* 31, no. 2 (March 1, 2021): 157–63. https://doi.org/10.1016/j.whi.2020.10.003.

Chapter 9

Bedsider. "All About Hormones!" *Bedsider*, January 27, 2014. https://www.bedsider.org/features/317-all-about-hormones.

Bedsider. "Video Reviews | Real Stories – Alyssa, 20, the Shot," *Bedsider*, January 6, 2010. https://www.bedsider.org/features/51-alyssa-20-the-shot.

Bedsider. "Video Reviews | Real Stories – Emily, 28, Sterilization," *Bedsider*, January 7, 2010. https://www.bedsider.org/birth-control/sterilization/reviews?feature=60&method=sterilization.

Bedsider. "Types of Birth Control," *Bedsider*, n.d. https://www.bedsider.org/birth-control

Callegari, Lisa S., Xinhua Zhao, Eleanor Bimla Schwarz, Elian Rosenfeld, Maria K. Mor, and Sonya Borrero. "Racial/Ethnic Differences in Contraceptive Preferences, Beliefs, and Self-efficacy Among Women Veterans," *American Journal of Obstetrics and Gynecology* 216, no. 5 (May 1, 2017): 504.e1–10. https://doi.org/10.1016/j.ajog.2016.12.178.

Centers for Disease Control and Prevention. "Management of Bleeding Irregularities While Using Contraception," *U.S. Selected Practice Recommendations for Contraceptive Use*, 2024. https://www.cdc.gov/contraception/media/pdfs/2024/07/management-during-contraception-508.pdf

Columbia University Irving Medical Center. "Personal Stories About Choosing Birth Control Methods," n.d. https://www.columbiadoctors.org/health-library/article/personal-stories-about-choosing-birth-control-methods/.

Columbia University Mailman School of Public Health. "Abstinence-Only Education Is a Failure," August 22, 2017. https://www.publichealth.columbia.edu/news/abstinence-only-education-failure.

Cooper, Danielle B., and Preeti Patel. "Oral Contraceptive Pills," StatPearls - NCBI Bookshelf, February 29, 2024. https://www.ncbi.nlm.nih.gov/books/NBK430882/.

Dehlendorf, Christine, Eric Vittinghoff, Judith Fitzpatrick, Edith Fox, Kelsey Holt, Reiley Reed, Maria Paula Campora, Abby Sokoloff, and Miriam Kuppermann. "A Decision Aid to Help Women Choose and Use a Method of Birth Control," *Patient-Centered Outcomes Research Institute (PCORI)*, October 4, 2019. https://doi.org/10.25302/10.2019.ce.13046874.

Frederiksen, Brittni, Usha Ranji, Michelle Long, Karen Diep, and Alina Salganicoff. "Contraception in the United States: A Closer Look at Experiences, Preferences, and Coverage," *KFF*, November 18, 2022. https://www.kff.org/womens-health-policy/report/contraception-in-the-united-states-a-closer-look-at-experiences-preferences-and-coverage/.

Jackson, Andrea V., Deborah Karasek, Christine Dehlendorf, and Diana Greene Foster. "Racial and Ethnic Differences in Women's Preferences for Features of Contraceptive Methods," *Contraception* 93, no. 5 (May 1, 2016): 406–11. https://doi.org/10.1016/j.contraception.2015.12.010.

Kaiser Family Foundation. "Emergency Contraception," *KFF*, August 4, 2022. https://www.kff.org/womens-health-policy/fact-sheet/emergency-contraception/

Marnach, Mary. "What Ovulation Signs Can I Watch for if I Want to Get Pregnant?" *Mayo Clinic*, n.d. https://www.mayoclinic.org/healthy-lifestyle/getting-pregnant/expert-answers/ovulation-signs/faq-20058000.

Mayo Clinic. "Delaying Your Period With Hormonal Birth Control," *Mayo Clinic*, December 2, 2022. https://www.mayoclinic.org/healthy-lifestyle/birth-control/in-depth/womens-health/art-20044044.

McGowan, Emma. "Why I Use a Diaphragm for Birth Control," *Bedsider*, November 5, 2019. https://www.bedsider.org/features/1345-why-i-use-a-diaphragm-for-birth-control.

National Survey of Family Growth. "Current Contraceptive Status," *National Center for Health Statistics* (NCHS), May 2021. https://www.cdc.gov/nchs/about/factsheets/factsheet-nsfg.htm.

Nguyen, A. T., Curtis, K. M., Tepper, N. K., et al. "U.S. Medical Eligibility Criteria for Contraceptive Use," *MMWR Recomm Report* 73, no. 4 (2024): 1–126. http://dx.doi.org/10.15585/mmwr.rr7304a1.

Planned Parenthood. "Birth Control," *Planned Parenthood*, n.d. https://www.plannedparenthood.org/learn/birth-control.

Planned Parenthood. "Breastfeeding," *Planned Parenthood*, n.d. https://www.plannedparenthood.org/learn/birth-control/breastfeeding.

Planned Parenthood. "Is It Unhealthy if You Skip Your Period While Using Mirena or Other Birth Control Methods?" *Planned Parenthood*, September 22, 2014. https://www.plannedparenthood.org/blog/is-it-unhealthy-if-you-skip-your-period-while-using-mirena-or-other-birth-control-methods.

Planned Parenthood. "What's The Best Birth Control Option While Breastfeeding?" *Planned Parenthood*, n.d. https://www.plannedparenthood.org/learn/birth-control/breastfeeding/whats-best-birth-control-option-while-breastfeeding.

Reproductive Health National Training Center. "Birth Control Methods Chart," *RHNTC*, July 2024. https://rhntc.org/resources/birth-control-methods-chart.

Reproductive Health National Training Center. "Breastfeeding and Contraception: Counseling Considerations Job Aid," April 2022. https://rhntc.org/resources/breastfeeding-and-contraception-counseling-considerations-job-aid.

Reproductive Health National Training Center. "Emergency Contraceptive (EC) Methods Table," January 2024. https://rhntc.org/resources/emergency-contraceptive-ec-methods-table.

Santelli, John, Stephanie Grilo, Laura Lindberg, Ilene Speizer, Amy Schalet, Jennifer Heitel, M. Heilbrunn, et al. "Abstinence-Only-Until-Marriage Policies and Programs: An Updated Position Paper of the Society for Adolescent Health and Medicine," *Journal of Adolescent Health* 61, no. 3 (September 1, 2017): 400–3. https://doi.org/10.1016/j.jadohealth.2017.06.001.

Trevino, Julissa. "Why My Mirena is My Ride or Die," Bedsider, *Bedsider*, October 8, 2019. https://www.bedsider.org/features/1335-why-my-mirena-is-my-ride-or-die.

Underhill, Kristen, Don Operario, and Paul Montgomery. "Abstinence-only Programs for HIV Infection Prevention in High-income Countries," *Cochrane Library*, October 17, 2007. https://doi.org/10.1002/14651858.cd005421.pub2.

University of California, San Francisco. "The Menstrual Cycle," *UCSF*, n.d. https://www.ucsfhealth.org/education/the-menstrual-cycle.

U.S. Food and Drug Administration. "FDA Allows Marketing of First Direct-to-Consumer App for Contraceptive Use to Prevent Pregnancy," *FDA*, August 10, 2018. https://www.fda.gov/news-events/press-announcements/fda-allows-marketing-first-direct-consumer-app-contraceptive-use-prevent-pregnancy.

U.S. Food and Drug Administration. "FDA Approves First Nonprescription Daily Oral Contraceptive," *FDA*, July 13, 2023. https://www.fda.gov/news-events/press-announcements/fda-approves-first-nonprescription-daily-oral-contraceptive.

Chapter 10

American Cancer Society. "Colorectal Cancer Facts & Figures 2020–2022," *Atlanta: American Cancer Society*, 2020. https://www.cancer.org/content/dam/cancer-org/research/cancer-facts-and-statistics/colorectal-cancer-facts-and-figures/colorectal-cancer-facts-and-figures-2020-2022.pdf.

American College of Obstetricians and Gynecologists. "Cervical Cancer Screening," *ACOG*, May 2021. https://www.acog.org/womens-health/faqs/cervical-cancer-screening.

American College of Obstetricians and Gynecologists. "Hormonal Contraception and Risk of Breast Cancer," *ACOG*, January 2018 (reaffirmed October 2023). https://www.acog.org/clinical/clinical-guidance/practice-advisory/articles/2018/01/hormonal-contraception-and-risk-of-breast-cancer.

American College of Obstetricians and Gynecologists. "Progestin-Only Hormonal Birth Control: Pill and Injection," *ACOG*, January 2023. https://www.acog.org/womens-health/faqs/progestin-only-hormonal-birth-control-pill-and-injection.

Armstrong, Carrie. "ACOG Guidelines on Noncontraceptive Uses of Hormonal Contraceptives," *American Family Physician* 82, no. 3. (August 1, 2010): 288–95. https://www.aafp.org/pubs/afp/issues/2010/0801/p288.html.

Arowojolu, Ayodele O., Maria F. Gallo, Laureen M. Lopez, David A. Grimes. "Combined Oral Contraceptive Pills for Treatment of Acne," *Cochrane Library*, July 11, 2012. https://www.cochranelibrary.com/cdsr/doi/10.1002/14651858.CD004425.pub6/full.

Asthana, Smita, Vishal Busa, and Satyanarayana Labani. "Oral Contraceptives Use and Risk of Cervical cancer—A Systematic Review &Amp; Meta-analysis," *European Journal of Obstetrics, Gynecology, and Reproductive Biology* 247 (April 1, 2020): 163–75. https://doi.org/10.1016/j.ejogrb.2020.02.014.

Bahamondes, Luis, M. Valeria Bahamondes, and Lee P. Shulman. "Non-contraceptive Benefits of Hormonal and Intrauterine Reversible Contraceptive Methods," *Human Reproduction Update* 21, no. 5 (June 1, 2015): 640–51. https://doi.org/10.1093/humupd/dmv023.

Beining, Robin M., Leslie K. Dennis, Elaine M. Smith, and Anuja Dokras. "Meta-Analysis of Intrauterine Device Use and Risk of Endometrial Cancer," *Annals of Epidemiology* 18, no. 6 (June 1, 2008): 492–9. https://doi.org/10.1016/j.annepidem.2007.11.011.

Benshushan, Abraham, Ora Paltiel, Nathan Rojansky, Amnon Brzezinski, and Neri Laufer. "IUD Use and the Risk of Endometrial Cancer," *European Journal of Obstetrics & Gynecology and Reproductive Biology* 105, no. 2 (November 1, 2002): 166–9. https://doi.org/10.1016/s0301-2115(02)00153-7.

Beral, V., R. Doll, C. Hermon, R. Peto, and G. Reeves. "Ovarian Cancer and Oral Contraceptives: Collaborative Reanalysis of Data From 45 Epidemiological Studies Including 23 257 Women With Ovarian Cancer and 87 303

Controls," *Lancet* 371, no. 9609 (January 1, 2008): 303–14. https://doi.org/10.1016/s0140-6736(08)60167-1.

Bosetti, Cristina, Francesca Bravi, Eva Negri, and Carlo La Vecchia. "Oral Contraceptives and Colorectal Cancer Risk: A Systematic Review and Meta-analysis," *Human Reproduction Update* 15, no. 5 (January 1, 2009): 489–98. https://doi.org/10.1093/humupd/dmp017.

Brabaharan, Sharmila, Sajesh K. Veettil, Jennifer E. Kaiser, Vrosha Rau Raja Rao, Rujira Wattanayingcharoenchai, Marikannan Maharajan, Putsarat Insin, et al. "Association of Hormonal Contraceptive Use With Adverse Health Outcomes," *JAMA Network Open* 5, no. 1 (January 14, 2022): e2143730. https://doi.org/10.1001/jamanetworkopen.2021.43730.

Burton, J. L., W. J. Cunliffe, Ilva Stafford, and Sam Shuster. "The Prevalence of Acne Vulgaris in Adolescence," *British Journal of Dermatology* 85, no. 2 (August 1, 1971): 119–26. https://doi.org/10.1111/j.1365-2133.1971.tb07195.x.

Centers for Disease Control and Prevention. "About Congenital Syphilis," *CDC*, April 8, 2024. https://www.cdc.gov/syphilis/about/about-congenital-syphilis.html.

Centers for Disease Control and Prevention. "About Genital Herpes," *CDC*, February 20, 2024. https://www.cdc.gov/herpes/about/index.html.

Centers for Disease Control and Prevention. "About Heavy Menstrual Bleeding," *CDC*, May 15, 2024. https://www.cdc.gov/female-blood-disorders/about/heavy-menstrual-bleeding.html.

Centers for Disease Control and Prevention. "About Sickle Cell Disease," *CDC*, May 15, 2024. https://www.cdc.gov/sickle-cell/about/.

Centers for Disease Control and Prevention. "Atlas Plus Charts: HIV Diagnoses," *CDC*, n.d. https://gis.cdc.gov/grasp/nchhstpatlas/charts.html.

Centers for Disease Control and Prevention. "Data and Statistics on Sickle Cell Disease," *CDC*, May 15, 2024. https://www.cdc.gov/sickle-cell/data/.

Centers for Disease Control and Prevention. "Fast Facts: HIV in the United States," *CDC*, April 22, 2024. https://www.cdc.gov/hiv/data-research/facts-stats/index.html

Centers for Disease Control and Prevention. "Incidence, Prevalence, and Cost of Sexually Transmitted Infections in the United States, 2018," *CDC*, March 8, 2024. https://www.cdc.gov/nchhstp-newsroom/factsheets/incidence-prevalence-cost-stis-in-us.html.

Centers for Disease Control and Prevention. "Management of Bleeding Irregularities While Using Contraception," *U.S. Selected Practice Recommendations for Contraceptive Use*, 2024. https://www.cdc.gov/contraception/media/pdfs/2024/07/management-during-contraception-508.pdf.

Centers for Disease Control and Prevention. "Screening Recommendations and Considerations Referenced in Treatment Guidelines and Original Sources," *CDC*, March 22, 2024. https://www.cdc.gov/std/treatment-guidelines/screening-recommendations.htm.

Centers for Disease Control and Prevention. "Sexually Transmitted Infections Surveillance, 2022," *CDC*, January 30, 2024. https://www.cdc.gov/std/statistics/2022/default.htm.

Centers for Disease Control and Prevention. "The State of STIs," *CDC*, April 3, 2024. https://www.cdc.gov/sti/php/communication-resources/the-state-of-stis.html.

Centers for Disease Control and Prevention. "Trichomoniasis," *CDC*, September 21, 2022. https://www.cdc.gov/std/treatment-guidelines/trichomoniasis.htm.

Centers for Disease Control and Prevention. "The Untreated Syphilis Study at Tuskegee Timeline," December 5, 2022. https://www.cdc.gov/tuskegee/timeline.htm.

Cleveland Clinic. "A Guide to Birth Control in Your 40s and 50s," *Cleveland Clinic*, May 11, 2023. https://health.clevelandclinic.org/birth-control-during-perimenopause.

Cleveland Clinic. "Premenstrual Dysphoric Disorder (PMDD)," *Cleveland Clinic*, n.d. https://my.clevelandclinic.org/health/diseases/9132-premenstrual-dysphoric-disorder-pmdd.

Colditz, G. A. "Oral Contraceptive Use and Mortality During 12 Years of Follow-Up: The Nurses' Health Study," *Annals of Internal Medicine* 120, no. 10 (May 15, 1994): 821. https://doi.org/10.7326/0003-4819-120-10-199405150-00002.

Costello, Michael F, Bhushan Shrestha, John Eden, Neil Johnson, and Lisa J Moran. "Insulin-sensitising Drugs Versus the Combined Oral Contraceptive Pill for Hirsutism, Acne and Risk of Diabetes, Cardiovascular Disease, and Endometrial Cancer in Polycystic Ovary Syndrome," *Cochrane Library*, January 24, 2007. https://doi.org/10.1002/14651858.cd005552.pub2.

Crowley, Jeffrey S., Amy B. Geller, and Sten H. Vermund. "Patterns and Drivers of STIs in the United States," *Sexually Transmitted Infections: Adopting a Sexual Health Paradigm - NCBI Bookshelf*, March 24, 2021. https://www.ncbi.nlm.nih.gov/books/NBK573159/.

Frederiksen, Brittni, Usha Ranji, Michelle Long, Karen Diep, and Alina Salganicoff. "Contraception in the United States: A Closer Look at Experiences, Preferences, and Coverage," *KFF*, November 18, 2022. https://www.kff.org/womens-health-policy/report/contraception-in-the-united-states-a-closer-look-at-experiences-preferences-and-coverage/.

Friberg, Britt, Ann Kristin Örnö, Annika Lindgren, and Stefan Lethagen. "Bleeding Disorders Among Young Women: A Population-based Prevalence Study," *Acta Obstetricia Et Gynecologica Scandinavica* 85, no. 2 (February 1, 2006): 200–6. https://doi.org/10.1080/00016340500342912.

Guttmacher Institute. "Contraceptive Use in the United States by Demographics," *Guttmacher Institute*, August 24, 2022. https://www.guttmacher.org/fact-sheet/contraceptive-use-united-states.

Hannaford, P. C, L. Iversen, T. V. Macfarlane, A. M. Elliott, V. Angus, and A. J. Lee. "Mortality Among Contraceptive Pill Users: Cohort Evidence From Royal College of General Practitioners' Oral Contraception Study," *BMJ* 340, no. 1 (March 11, 2010): c927. https://doi.org/10.1136/bmj.c927.

HIV.gov. "Pre-Exposure Prophylaxis," June 27, 2024. https://www.hiv.gov/hiv-basics/hiv-prevention/using-hiv-medication-to-reduce-risk/pre-exposure-prophylaxis.

Hubacher, David, and David A. Grimes. "Noncontraceptive Health Benefits of Intrauterine Devices: A Systematic Review," *Obstetrical & Gynecological Survey* 57, no. 2 (February 1, 2002): 120–8. https://doi.org/10.1097/00006254-200202000-00024.

Jones, Rachel K. "Beyond Birth Control: The Overlooked Benefits Of Oral Contraceptive Pills," *Guttmacher Institute*, November 2011. https://www.guttmacher.org/sites/default/files/pdfs/pubs/Beyond-Birth-Control.pdf.

Ju, Hong, Mark Jones, and Gita Mishra. "The Prevalence and Risk Factors of Dysmenorrhea," *Epidemiologic Reviews* 36, no. 1 (November 26, 2013): 104–13. https://doi.org/10.1093/epirev/mxt009.

Kaiser Family Foundation. "KFF Poll: Most Americans Are Unaware of How Common STIs Are Among Adults and That Rates Are Rising," *KFF*, February 18, 2020 https://www.kff.org/womens-health-policy/press-release/kff-poll-most-americans-are-unaware-of-how-common-stis-are-among-adults-and-that-rates-are-rising/.

Kirzinger Ashley, Cailey Muñana, Mollyann Brodie, Brittni Frederiksen, Gabriela Weigel, Usha Ranji, and Alina Salganicoff. "Public Knowledge and Attitudes About Sexually Transmitted Infections: KFF Polling and Policy Insights," *KFF*, February 18, 2020. https://www.kff.org/womens-health-policy/issue-brief/public-knowledge-and-attitudes-about-sexually-transmitted-infections/.

Latthe, Pallavi, Manish Latthe, Lale Say, Metin Gülmezoglu, and Khalid S. Khan. "WHO Systematic Review of Prevalence of Chronic Pelvic Pain: A Neglected Reproductive Health Morbidity," *BMC Public Health* 6, no. 1 (July 6, 2006): 177. https://doi.org/10.1186/1471-2458-6-177.

LeDuc, Maggi. "How Birth Control Can Help With Gender Dysphoria," *Power to Decide*. August 10, 2020. https://powertodecide.org/news/how-birth-control-can-help-gender-dysphoria.

Leigh E. Szucs et al., "Condom and Contraceptive Use Among Sexually Active High School Students — Youth Risk Behavior Survey, United States, 2019," *MMWR Supplements* 69, no. 1 (August 21, 2020): 11–18. https://doi.org/10.15585/mmwr.su6901a2.

Lethaby, Anne, Munawar Hussain, Josephine R. Rishworth, and Margaret C. Rees. "Progesterone or Progestogen-releasing Intrauterine Systems for Heavy Menstrual Bleeding," *Cochrane Library*, April 30, 2015. https://doi.org/10.1002/14651858.cd002126.pub3.

Lowe, Richard F., and Ndola Prata. "Hemoglobin and Serum Ferritin Levels in Women Using Copper-releasing or Levonorgestrel-releasing Intrauterine Devices: A Systematic Review," *Contraception* 87, no. 4 (April 1, 2013): 486–96. https://doi.org/10.1016/j.contraception.2012.09.025.

Mayo Clinic. "Heavy Menstrual Bleeding," *Mayo Clinic*, August 30, 2023. https://www.mayoclinic.org/diseases-conditions/menorrhagia/symptoms-causes/syc-20352829.

Mayo Clinic. "Syphilis," *Mayo Clinic*, July 20, 2024. https://www.mayoclinic.org/diseases-conditions/syphilis/symptoms-causes/syc-20351756.

Minalt, Nicole, Amy Caldwell, Grace M. Yedlicka, Sophia Joseph, Sharon E. Robertson, Lisa M. Landrum, and Jeffrey F. Peipert. "Association Between Intrauterine Device Use and Endometrial, Cervical, and Ovarian Cancer: An Expert Review," *American Journal of Obstetrics and Gynecology* 229, no. 2 (August 1, 2023): 93–100. https://doi.org/10.1016/j.ajog.2023.03.039.

National Academies Press. "Contraceptive Benefits and Risks," *Contraception and Reproduction: Health Consequences for Women and Children in the Developing World*, 1989. https://www.ncbi.nlm.nih.gov/books/NBK235069/.

National Cancer Institute. "HPV Vaccination," *NCI*, March 2024. https://progressreport.cancer.gov/prevention/hpv_immunization.

National Cancer Institute. "Human Papillomavirus (HPV) Vaccines," *NCI*, May 25, 2021. https://www.cancer.gov/about-cancer/causes-prevention/risk/hormones/oral-contraceptives-fact-sheet.

National Cancer Institute. "Oral Contraceptives and Cancer Risk," *NCI*, February 22, 2018. https://www.cancer.gov/about-cancer/causes-prevention/risk/hormones/oral-contraceptives-fact-sheet.

National Cancer Institute Surveillance, Epidemiology, and End Results (SEER) Program. "Cancer Stat Facts: Ovarian Cancer," *SEER*, n.d. https://seer.cancer.gov/statfacts/html/ovary.html.

National Cancer Institute Surveillance, Epidemiology, and End Results (SEER) Program. "Cancer Stat Facts: Uterine Cancer," *SEER*, n.d. https://seer.cancer.gov/statfacts/html/corp.html.

National Center for Quality Assurance. "Lead Screening in Children (LSC)," *NCQA*, n.d. https://www.ncqa.org/hedis/measures/lead-screening-in-children/.

National Coalition of STD Directors. "Out-of-Control STI Epidemic Continues to Put Lives at Risk," January 30, 2024. https://www.ncsddc.org/out-of-control-sti-epidemic-continues-to-put-lives-at-risk/.

National Coalition of STD Directors. "U.S STI Rates Hit Another High," April 11, 2023. https://www.ncsddc.org/u-s-sti-rates-hit-another-high/.

National Heart, Lung, and Blood Institute. "What Is Venous Thromboembolism?" *NHLBI*, September 19, 2022. https://www.nhlbi.nih.gov/health/venous-thromboembolism.

National Survey of Family Growth. "NSFG - Listing C - Key Statistics From the National Survey of Family Growth," *National Center for Health Statistics (NCHS)*, n.d. https://www.cdc.gov/nchs/nsfg/key_statistics/c-keystat.htm#contraception.

National Women's Law Center. "Our Fight in the Supreme Court Includes Your Stories About Birth Control," April 9, 2020 https://nwlc.org/our-fight-in-the-supreme-court-includes-your-stories-about-birth-control/.

Nguyen, A. T., Curtis, K. M., Tepper, N. K., et al. "U.S. Medical Eligibility Criteria for Contraceptive Use," *MMWR Recomm Report* 73, no. 4 (2024): 1–126. http://dx.doi.org/10.15585/mmwr.rr7304a1.

Office on Women's Health. "Endometriosis," February 22, 2021. https://www.womenshealth.gov/a-z-topics/endometriosis.

Park, Ina. *Strange Bedfellows: Adventures in the Science, History, and Surprising Secrets of STDs*. Flatiron Books, February 2, 2021.

Parker, Ma, Ae Sneddon, and P. Arbon. "The Menstrual Disorder of Teenagers (MDOT) Study: Determining Typical Menstrual Patterns and Menstrual Disturbance in a Large Population-based Study of Australian Teenagers," *BJOG* 117, no. 2 (December 9, 2009): 185–92. https://doi.org/10.1111/j.1471-0528.2009.02407.x.

Planned Parenthood Action Fund. "Stories: The Benefits of Birth Control," *Planned Parenthood*, n.d. https://www.plannedparenthoodaction.org/issues/birth-control/birth-control-stories.

Planned Parenthood. "The Birth Control Pill: A History," *Planned Parenthood*, 2015. https://www.plannedparenthood.org/files/1514/3518/7100/Pill_History_FactSheet.pdf.

Power to Decide. "2023 #ThxBirthControl Survey Data," November 2023. https://powertodecide.org/what-we-do/information/resource-library/2023-thxbirthcontrol-survey-data.

Rodrigues, Ana Cláudia, Sónia Gala, Ângela Neves, Conceição Pinto, Cláudia Meirelles, Cristina Frutuoso, Maria Elisete Vítor. "[Dysmenorrhea in Adolescents and Young Adults: Prevalence, Related Factors and Limitations in Daily Living]," *Acta Med Port* 2 (December 31 2011): 383–88.

Roe, Andrea H., Deborah A. Bartz, Pamela S. Douglas. "Combined Estrogen-Progestin Contraception: Side Effects and Health Concerns," *UpToDate*, October 23, 2023. https://www.uptodate.com/contents/combined-estrogen-progestin-contraception-side-effects-and-health-concerns#H2769334788.

Schindler, Adolf E. "Non-Contraceptive Benefits of Oral Hormonal Contraceptives," *International Journal of Endocrinology and Metabolism* 11, no. 1 (December 21, 2012). https://doi.org/10.5812/ijem.4158.

Słopień, Radosław, Ewa Milewska, Piotr Rynio, and Błażej Męczekalski. "Use of Oral Contraceptives for Management of Acne Vulgaris and Hirsutism in Women of Reproductive and Late Reproductive Age," *Menopausal Review* 17, no. 1 (January 1, 2018): 1–4. https://doi.org/10.5114/pm.2018.74895.

Soini, Tuuli, Ritva Hurskainen, Seija Grénman, Johanna Mäenpää, Jorma Paavonen, and Eero Pukkala. "Cancer Risk in Women Using the Levonorgestrel-Releasing Intrauterine System in Finland," *Obstetrics and Gynecology* 124, no. 2 (August 1, 2014): 292–9. https://doi.org/10.1097/aog.0000000000000356.

Teal, Stephanie, and Alison Edelman. "Contraception Selection, Effectiveness, and Adverse Effects," *JAMA* 326, no. 24 (December 28, 2021): 2507. https://doi.org/10.1001/jama.2021.21392.

Tuesley, Karen, Katrina Spilsbury, Sallie-Anne Pearson et al. "Long-acting, progestin-based contraceptives and risk of breast, gynecological, and other cancers," *J Natl Cancer Inst.* 117, no. 5 (January 14 2025): 1046-1055. https://doi.org/10.1093/jnci/djae282.

U.S Department of Health and Human Services. "Sexually Transmitted Infections National Strategic Plan for the United States | 2021–2025," *Washington, DC*, 2020. https://www.hhs.gov/sites/default/files/STI-National-Strategic-Plan-2021-2025.pdf.

Vessey, Martin, Rosemary Painter, and David Yeates. "Mortality in Relation to Oral Contraceptive Use and Cigarette Smoking," *The Lancet* 362, no. 9379 (July 1, 2003): 185–91. https://doi.org/10.1016/s0140-6736(03)13907-4.

Westhoff, Carolyn L, Stephen Heartwell, Sharon Edwards, Mimi Zieman, Gretchen Stuart, Carrie Cwiak, Anne Davis, Tina Robilotto, Linda Cushman, and Debra Kalmuss. "Oral Contraceptive Discontinuation: Do Side Effects

Matter?" *American Journal of Obstetrics and Gynecology* 196, no. 4 (April 1, 2007): 412.e1–7. https://doi.org/10.1016/j.ajog.2006.12.015.

Weyand, Angela C., Alexander Chaitoff, Gary L. Freed, Michelle Sholzberg, Sung Won Choi, and Patrick T. McGann. "Prevalence of Iron Deficiency and Iron-Deficiency Anemia in US Females Aged 12–21 Years, 2003–2020," *JAMA* 329, no. 24 (June 27, 2023): 2191. https://doi.org/10.1001/jama.2023.8020.

Workowski, Kimberly A., Laura H. Bachmann, Philip A. Chan, Christine M. Johnston, Christina A. Muzny, Ina Park, Hilary Reno, Jonathan M. Zenilman, and Gail A. Bolan. "Sexually Transmitted Infections Treatment Guidelines, 2021," *Morbidity and Mortality Weekly Report. Recommendations and Reports* 70, no. 4 (July 23, 2021): 1–187. https://doi.org/10.15585/mmwr.rr7004a1.

World Health Organization. "Endometriosis," *WHO*, March 24, 2023. https://www.who.int/news-room/fact-sheets/detail/endometriosis.

World Health Organization. "WHO Statement on Menstrual Health and Rights," *WHO*, June 22, 2022. https://www.who.int/news/item/22-06-2022-who-statement-on-menstrual-health-and-rights.

Yale Medicine. "Endometrial Hyperplasia," n.d. *Yale Medicine*, https://www.yalemedicine.org/conditions/endometrial-hyperplasia.

Zabiegalski, Robin. "I Have a Chronic Illness and Birth Control Changed My Life," *Bedsider*, September 10, 2019. https://www.bedsider.org/features/1324-i-have-a-chronic-illness-and-birth-control-changed-my-life.

Chapter 11

Abma, Joyce C., and Gladys Martinez. "Teenagers in the United States: Sexual Activity, Contraceptive Use, and Childbearing, 2015–2019," *CDC*, December 14, 2023. https://www.cdc.gov/nchs/data/nhsr/nhsr196.pdf.

Association of American Medical Colleges. "2022 Physician Specialty Data Report – Executive Summary," *AAMC*, January 2023. https://www.aamc.org/media/63371/download?attachment.

Association of American Medical Colleges. "Figure 12. Percentage of U.S. Medical School Graduates by Sex, Academic Years 1980–1981 Through 2018–2019," *AAMC*, n.d. https://www.aamc.org/data-reports/workforce/data/figure-12-percentage-us-medical-school-graduates-sex-academic-years-1980-1981-through-2018-2019.

American Bar Association. "ABA Profile of the Legal Profession – Growth of the Legal Profession," *ABA*, n.d. https://www.abalegalprofile.com/demographics.html.

American Dental Association. "Dental Education," *ADA*, n.d. https://www.ada.org/resources/research/health-policy-institute/dental-education.

Bailey, Martha J. "Fifty Years of Family Planning: New Evidence on the Long-Run Effects of Increasing Access to Contraception," *Brookings Papers on Economic Activity* 2013, no. 1 (March 1, 2013): 341–409. https://doi.org/10.1353/eca.2013.0001.

Brenan, Megan. "Women Still Handle Main Household Tasks in U.S," *Gallup*, January 29, 2020. https://news.gallup.com/poll/283979/women-handle-main-household-tasks.aspx.

Center on the Economics of Reproductive Health. "The Economic Effects of Contraceptive Access: A Review of the Evidence," *Institute for Women's Policy Research*, 2019. Washington, DC. https://iwpr.org/wp-content/uploads/2020/07/B381_Contraception-Access_Final.pdf.

Centers for Disease Control and Prevention. "Achievements in Public Health, 1900-1999: Family Planning," *MMWR* 28 no. 47 (December 3, 1999): 1073–80. https://www.cdc.gov/mmwr/preview/mmwrhtml/mm4847a1.htm.

Centers for Disease Control and Prevention. "Ten Great Public Health Achievements -- United States, 1900–1999," *MMWR* 48 no. 12 (April 2, 1999): 241–3. https://www.cdc.gov/mmwr/preview/mmwrhtml/00056796.htm.

Columbia University Center on Poverty and Social Policy. "Anti-Poverty Policies and Programs — Columbia University Center on Poverty and Social Policy," n.d. https://www.povertycenter.columbia.edu/policies-and-programs.

DaVanzo, Julie, and David M. Adamson. "Family Planning in Developing Countries: An Unfinished Success Story," *Rand*, 1998. https://www.rand.org/pubs/issue_papers/IP176.html.

Duncan, Greg J., and Harry J. Holzer. "Policies That Reduce Intergenerational Poverty," *Brookings*, October 17, 2023. https://www.brookings.edu/articles/policies-that-reduce-intergenerational-poverty/.

Finlay, Jocelyn E., and Marlene A. Lee. "Identifying Causal Effects of Reproductive Health Improvements on Women's Economic Empowerment Through the Population Poverty Research Initiative," *The Milbank Quarterly* 96, no. 2 (June 1, 2018): 300–22. https://doi.org/10.1111/1468-0009.12326.

HHS Office of Population Affairs. "Trends in Teen Pregnancy and Childbearing," n.d. https://opa.hhs.gov/adolescent-health/reproductive-health-and-teen-pregnancy/trends-teen-pregnancy-and-childbearing.

Jalanko, Eerika, Frida Gyllenberg, Nikolas Krstic, Mika Gissler, and Oskari Heikinheimo. "Municipal Contraceptive Services, Socioeconomic Status and Teenage Pregnancy in Finland: A Longitudinal Study," *BMJ Open* 11, no. 2 (February 1, 2021): e043092. https://doi.org/10.1136/bmjopen-2020-043092.

Joint Economic Committee. "The Economic Benefits of Birth Control and Access to Family Planning," *JEC*, Updated February, 2020. https://www.jec.senate.gov/public/_cache/files/bb400414-8dee-4e39-abd3-c2460fd30e7d/the-economic-benefits-of-birth-control-and-access-to-family-planning.pdf.

Katz, Elizabeth D., Kyle Rozema, and Sarath Sanga. "Women in U.S. Law Schools, 1948–2021," *The Journal of Legal Analysis* 15, no. 1 (August 21, 2023): 48–78. https://doi.org/10.1093/jla/laad005.

Kochhar, Rakesh "The Enduring Grip of the Gender Pay Gap," *Pew Research Center*, March 1, 2023. https://www.pewresearch.org/social-trends/2023/03/01/the-enduring-grip-of-the-gender-pay-gap/.

Livingston, Gretchen, and Deja Thomas. "Why is the Teen Birth Rate Falling?" *Pew Research Center*, August 2, 2019. https://www.pewresearch.org/short-reads/2019/08/02/why-is-the-teen-birth-rate-falling/.

Planned Parenthood. "Birth Control Has Expanded Opportunity for Women," June 2015. https://www.plannedparenthood.org/files/1614/3275/8659/BC_factsheet_may2015_updated_1.pdf.

Planned Parenthood. "The Birth Control Pill: A History," 2015. https://www.plannedparenthood.org/files/1514/3518/7100/Pill_History_FactSheet.pdf.

Planned Parenthood. "*Griswold v. Connecticut* – The Impact of Legal Birth Control and the Challenges that Remain," May 2015. https://cdn.plannedparenthood.org/uploads/filer_public/b6/7c/b67c1da4-c40a-4d0f-90af-952fdbf11fbf/factsheet_griswold_may2015_r2.pdf.

Planned Parenthood. "Reducing Teenage Pregnancy," June 2014. https://www.plannedparenthood.org/uploads/filer_public/94/d7/94d748c6-5be0-4765-9d38-b1b90d16a254/reducing_teen_pregnancy.pdf.

Power to Decide. "Contraceptive Deserts," n.d. https://powertodecide.org/what-we-do/contraceptive-deserts.

Sonfield, Adam, Kinsey Hasstedt, Megan L. Kavanaugh, and Ragnar Anderson. "The Social and Economic Benefits of Women's Ability to Determine Whether and When to Have Children," March 2013. https://www.guttmacher.org/sites/default/files/pdfs/pubs/social-economic-benefits.pdf.

Statista. "Life Expectancy (From Birth) In the United States, From 1860–2020," July 4, 2024. https://www.statista.com/statistics/1040079/life-expectancy-united-states-all-time/.

Statista. "Percentage of the U.S Population Who Have Completed Four Years of College or More From 1940–2022, by Gender," July 5, 2024. https://www.statista.com/statistics/184272/educational-attainment-of-college-diploma-or-higher-by-gender/.

United Nations. "World Family Planning 2022," Department of Economic and Social Affairs, Population Division. New York, 2022. https://www.un.org/

development/desa/pd/sites/www.un.org.development.desa.pd/files/files/documents/2023/Feb/undesa_pd_2022_world-family-planning.pdf.

University of California San Francisco. "The Person-Centered Contraceptive Counseling (PCCC) Measure," *Person-Centered Reproductive Health Program*, n.d. https://pcccmeasure.ucsf.edu/.

University of California San Francisco. "Self-Identified Need for Contraception (SINC) Implementation Guidance," *Person-Centered Reproductive Health Program*, n.d. https://pcrhp.ucsf.edu/SINC.

U.S Department of Health and Human Services. "HHS, DOL, and Treasury Issue Guidance Regarding Birth Control Coverage," July 28, 2022. https://www.hhs.gov/about/news/2022/07/28/hhs-dol-treasury-issue-guidance-regarding-birth-control-coverage.html.

World Economic Forum. "The Economic Benefits of Family Planning," *WEF*, July 26, 2018. https://www.weforum.org/agenda/2018/07/the-economic-benefits-of-family-planning/.

Youth.gov. "The Adverse Effects of Teen Pregnancy," n.d. https://youth.gov/youth-topics/pregnancy-prevention/adverse-effects-teen-pregnancy.

Chapter 12

American College of Obstetricians and Gynecologists. "Access to Contraception," *Committee on Health Care for Underserved Women, ACOG*, 2015 (reaffirmed 2022). https://www.acog.org/clinical/clinical-guidance/committee-opinion/articles/2015/01/access-to-contraception.

Anderson, Deborah J., and Daniel S. Johnston. "A Brief History and Future Prospects of Contraception," *Science* 380, no. 6641 (April 14, 2023): 154–8. https://doi.org/10.1126/science.adf9341.

Baker, Courtney C., and Melissa J. Chen. "New Contraception Update — Annovera, Phexxi, Slynd, and Twirla," *Current Obstetrics and Gynecology Reports* 11, no. 1 (January 6, 2022): 21–7. https://doi.org/10.1007/s13669-021-00321-4.

Callahan, Rebecca L., Neha J. Mehta, Kavita Nanda, and Gregory S. Kopf. "The New Contraceptive Revolution: Developing Innovative Products Outside of Industry," *Biology of Reproduction* 103, no. 2 (May 9, 2020): 157–66. https://doi.org/10.1093/biolre/ioaa067.

Colarossi, Jessica. "A New Breed of Nonhormonal Birth Control," *Boston University*, March 20, 2023. https://www.bu.edu/articles/2022/new-nonhormonal-birth-control/.

Daniels, Kimberly, and Joyce C. Abma. "Contraceptive Methods Women Have Ever Used: United States, 2015–2019," *National Health Statistics Reports*, December 14, 2023. https://www.cdc.gov/nchs/data/nhsr/nhsr195.pdf.

Eunice Kennedy Shriver National Institute of Child Health and Human Development. "Contraceptive Development Research Center Program (CDRCP)," May 10, 2023. https://www.nichd.nih.gov/research/supported/cdrcp.

Eunice Kennedy Shriver National Institute of Child Health and Human Development. "Contraceptive Research Branch (CRB)," March 18, 2024. https://www.nichd.nih.gov/about/org/der/branches/crb.

FHI 360. "Calliope, the Contraceptive Pipeline Database," *Contraceptive Technology Innovation (CTI) Exchange*. https://pipeline.ctiexchange.org/.

FHI 360. "FHI 360 Conducting Trial for Casea S, a Biodegradable Contraceptive Implant – FHI 360," *FHI*, February 20, 2024. https://www.fhi360.org/articles/fhi-360-conducting-trial-casea-s-biodegradable-contraceptive-implant/.

Frederiksen, Brittni, Usha Ranji, Michelle Long, Karen Diep, and Alina Salganicoff. "Contraception in the United States: A Closer Look at Experiences, Preferences, and Coverage," *KFF*, November 18, 2022. https://www.kff.org/womens-health-policy/report/contraception-in-the-united-states-a-closer-look-at-experiences-preferences-and-coverage/.

Guttmacher Institute. "Pharmacist-Prescribed Contraceptives," *Guttmacher Institute*, August 31, 2023. https://www.guttmacher.org/state-policy/explore/pharmacist-prescribed-contraceptives.

Haddad, Lisa B., John W. Townsend, and Regine Sitruk-Ware, "Contraceptive Technologies: Looking Ahead to New Approaches to Increase Options for Family Planning," *Clinical Obstetrics & Gynecology* 64, no. 3 (May 11, 2021): 435–48. https://doi.org/10.1097/grf.0000000000000628.

Hanaphy, Paul. "PharmED Backed by USAID to 3D Print Less-Intrusive Contraceptives for Women," *Printing Industry*, March 15, 2022. https://3dprintingindustry.com/news/pharme3d-backed-by-usaid-to-3d-print-less-intrusive-contraceptives-for-women-206073/.

National Survey of Family Growth. "NSFG - Listing C - Key Statistics From the National Survey of Family Growth," *National Center for Health Statistics (NCHS)*, n.d. https://www.cdc.gov/nchs/nsfg/key_statistics/c-keystat.htm#contraception.

Oregon Health & Science University. "Family Planning Program Research," *OHSU*, n.d. https://www.ohsu.edu/school-of-medicine/ob-gyn/family-planning-program-research.

Patil, Eva, and Jeffrey T. Jensen. "Update on Permanent Contraception Options for Women," *Current Opinion in Obstetrics & Gynecology* 27, no. 6 (December 1, 2015): 465–70. https://doi.org/10.1097/gco.0000000000000213.

Piper, Kelsey. "How Billionaire Philanthropy Provides Reproductive Health Care When Politicians Won't," *Vox*, September 17, 2019. https://www.vox.com/future-perfect/2019/9/17/20754970/billionaire-philanthropy-reproductive-health-care-politics.

Population Council. "The Dapivirine-Levonorgestrel Vaginal Ring for HIV Prevention and Contraception," *Population Council*, n.d. https://popcouncil.org/project/the-dapivirine-levonorgestrel-vaginal-ring-for-hiv-prevention-and-contraception/.

Population Council. "Dual Prevention Pill for the Prevention of HIV and Unintended Pregnancy," *Population Council*, n.d. https://popcouncil.org/project/dual-prevention-pill-for-the-prevention-of-hiv-and-unintended-pregnancy/.

Population Council. "International Committee for Contraception Research (ICCR)," *Population Council*, n.d. https://popcouncil.org/project/the-international-committee-for-contraception-research/

Population Council. "Nestorone®/Testosterone Transdermal Gel for Male Contraception," *Population Council*, n.d. https://popcouncil.org/project/nestorone-testosterone-transdermal-gel-for-male-contraception/.

Population Council. "Nonhormonal Contraceptive Multipurpose Prevention Technology Containing Q-Griffithsin," *Population Council*, n.d. https://popcouncil.org/project/non-hormonal-contraceptive-multipurpose-prevention-technology-mpt-containing-q-griffithsin/.

Population Council. "Products in Development," *Population Council*, n.d. https://popcouncil.org/cbr-products-in-development/.

United Nations. "World Family Planning 2022," *Department of Economic and Social Affairs, Population Division*. New York, 2022. https://www.un.org/development/desa/pd/sites/www.un.org.development.desa.pd/files/files/documents/2023/Feb/undesa_pd_2022_world-family-planning.pdf.

University of Texas at Austin. "PharmE3D Labs Receive Federal Funding for 3D Printed Contraception | College of Pharmacy," March 14, 2022. https://pharmacy.utexas.edu/node/1247.

U.S Food and Drug Administration. "Establishing Effectiveness and Safety for Hormonal Drug Products Intended to Prevent Pregnancy Guidance for Industry – Draft Guidance," *Center for Drug Evaluation and Research (CDER)*, July 2019. https://www.fda.gov/media/128792/download.

U.S Food and Drug Administration. "FDA Approves New Vaginal Ring for One Year of Birth Control," *FDA*, August 10, 2018. https://www.fda.gov/news

-events/press-announcements/fda-approves-new-vaginal-ring-one-year-birth-control.

Vogelsong, Kirsten. "New Contraceptive Technologies 2024: Investment in New Contraceptives for Women," *Bill & Melinda Gates Foundation*, September 26, 2023. https://www.gatesfoundation.org/ideas/articles/why-we-must-invest-in-new-womens-contraceptive-options.

Zhu, Baolin, Yifan Chen, Wenjie Lu, Qing Zhang, Song Gao, Lingfeng Sun, Shengqi Chen, and Rongfeng Hu. "A Biodegradable Long-term Contraceptive Implant With Steady Levonorgestrel Release Based on PLGA Microspheres Embedded in PCL-coated Implant," *Journal of Drug Delivery Science and Technology* 67 (January 1, 2022): 102955. https://doi.org/10.1016/j.jddst.2021.102955.

Chapter 13

Felix, Mabel Laurie Sobel, and Alina Salganicoff. "The Right to Contraception: State and Federal Actions, Misinformation, and the Courts," *KFF*, May 28, 2024. https://www.kff.org/womens-health-policy/issue-brief/the-right-to-contraception-state-and-federal-actions-misinformation-and-the-courts/.

HHS Office of Population Affairs. "Title X Program Funding History," *HHS*, n.d. https://opa.hhs.gov/grant-programs/archive/title-x-program-archive/title-x-program-funding-history.

Hill, Latoya, Samantha Artiga, and Anthony Damico. "Health Coverage by Race and Ethnicity, 2010–2022," *KFF*, January 11, 2024. https://www.kff.org/racial-equity-and-health-policy/issue-brief/health-coverage-by-race-and-ethnicity/.

Office of the Assistant Secretary for Planning and Evaluation. "National Uninsured Rate Reaches an All-Time Low in Early 2023," August 3, 2023. https://aspe.hhs.gov/reports/national-uninsured-rate-reaches-all-time-low-early-2023.

SisterSong. "Reproductive Justice," n.d. https://www.sistersong.net/reproductive-justice.

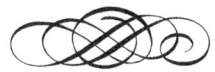

Index

abortion
    CHOICE Study results   109–10
    Gag Rule   55
    legality   5, 9–12, 48–49 (*see also Roe v. Wade*)
    and religion   39
    and Ronald Reagan   53–5
abstinence
    method   139–40, 145
    periodic   23–4, 37, 42
    postpartum   24
    promotion of   54
abstinence-only sex education   54, 57
access barriers   117–22
acne
    as a noncontraceptive benefit   133, 154–5, 160
    as a side effect   66
Affordable Care Act (ACA)   31, 111, 119, 126, 143, 176, 187
Alabama Supreme Court   6–7
American Birth Control League   76
American Medical Association   41, 47, 104
Ancient Egypt   18–20
Ancient Greece   16, 20–1

anemia   133, 153, 160
Aristotle   20
Ayurveda   22–3
azoospermia   64, 71

basal body temperature   25, 141–2
Bill & Melinda Gates Foundation   62, 185
birth spacing   21, 24, 36
Black Death (bubonic plague)   40
bleeding
    breakthrough   83, 130, 151, 154–8, 163
    heavy   151–5, 160
    lighter (as a side effect of birth control)   129–33, 149, 152–5, 163
    spotting (*see* bleeding; breakthrough)
    withdrawal   132
breastfeeding   35, 129, 132, 142, *see also* lactational amenorrhea method
Buck, Carrie   91–3
Buck v. Bell   92–3
Bush, George Herbert Walker (President)   52–3

Caesar, Julius   21
cancer
  breast   159
  cervical   159–61
  colorectal   149, 160, 163
  gynecological   149–50, 160, 163
  ovarian   149–50, 160, 163
  uterine   149–50, 160, 163
Casti Connubii   37
Catholicism, *see* religion
Centers for Disease Control and Prevention (CDC)   153, 158, 161–2, 165–6
cervical mucus   24–5, 83, 133
Chang, Min-Chueh Dr.   78–80
characteristics of birth control methods (table)   138–9
China's one-child policy   97
Clement of Alexandria (theologian)   37
Cleopatra   18
clinical trials   65–71, 183, *see also* Puerto Rico pill trials; US Food and Drug Administration
college enrollment   169–71
combined hormonal contraceptive   132–3, 138, 148–61
comprehensive sex education   57, 123, 168
Comstock, Anthony (and related Comstock laws)   45–9, 58, 75–81
condom
  coercion   122
  future   179–82
  historical use and development   20, 27, 43–7
  latex   61

  modern   60–3, 136, 139, 145
  prevalence   4, 38, 57
  for prevention of STIs   3, 136, 160–3
continuous use   132–4
Contraceptive CHOICE Project   109–11
Contraceptive Knowledge Assessment   28–30

Dalkon Shield   68–9, 105, 108
Darwin, Charles (Scientist)   90
Declaration of Helsinki   65–6
Depo-Provera, *see* injection
diaphragm
  as a birth control method   134–5, 138, 142, 145
  history of   47, 75–8
Dobbs v. Jackson Women's Health Organization   9–13, 122–3
douching syringes   42–3

Ebers Papyrus   19
economic benefits   165–76
Eisenhower, Dwight David (President)   51
Eisenstadt v. Baird   47–9
emergency contraception   4, 11–12, 129–30, 137, 139, 145
endometriosis   151–2, 160
Enovid   80–5, 102
enslaved people   24, 103–5, 112
eugenics   76, 90–9

family gap   172
family planning (term)   51–2
fast-dissolving insert   180
fertility awareness method (FAM)   4, 25, 139–42
foreign aid for family planning   51–6

Galton, Francis 90–1
gender dysphoria 3, 156–7
gender equality 165–76
gender pay gap 171–3
Goodyear, Charles 43
Grady Clinic 102
Grant, Ulysses S. (President) 46
Griswold v. Connecticut 47–9, 167–8

herbal remedies (historical) 20–8, 42
Hertwig, Oscar (Scientist) 18
Hippocrates 27
honey 20, 22
hormone safety 133, 142
Human Betterment Leagues 94–5
human immunodeficiency virus (HIV) 136–7, 162, 179–81
human papillomavirus (HPV) 159–62
Humanae Vitae (Of Human Life) 38, 53, 81
hysteria 21

immigrant 74, 92, 96, 112
implant, contraceptive
  access barriers 121
  benefits and side effects 148, 154, 157–60
  as a birth control method 126, 130–1, 138
  breastfeeding 142
  future 177–8, 183
  historical 108–13, 168
  Norplant controversy 105–8
  prevalence 4, 111
infant mortality 26, 166
injection (birth control shot)
  benefits and side effects 148, 154, 160

  as a birth control method 130–1, 138
  breastfeeding and 142
  future 180–2
  historical 89–90, 101–5
  for males 64, 70–1
  prevalence 4
insurance coverage and status, *see also* Affordable Care Act
  access barriers 11, 117–24
  birth control use by insurance status 2–4, 188
  Norplant controversy 107
  sterilization 99
  Title X 86
intrauterine device (IUD), *see also* Dalkon Shield
  access barriers 12, 117–24
  benefits and side effects 148–54, 160
  as a birth control method 128–33, 138
  breastfeeding and 142
  emergency contraception 129–30, 137
  future 178–84
  historical 90, 96, 108–13, 168
  prevalence 4, 168
in vitro fertilization (IVF) 6–9

Johnson, Lyndon B. (President) 52, 85

Kahun Gynaecological Papyrus 19
Kama Sutra 34
Kyleena 129, *see also* IUD

lactational amenorrhea method (LAM) 21, 23–4, 36, 142
Lee, Minnie 89–90, 93–7, 101
Liletta 129, *see also* IUD

long-acting reversible contraception 108–13, see also IUD; implant
Long-Acting Reversible Contraception Statement of Principles 111

Male Contraceptive Initiative 3, 69
male contraceptives 59–72, see also condom; vasectomy; withdrawal
Malthus, Thomas (Economist) 90
maternal morality 26, 166
McCormick, Katharine Dexter 74, 77–80, 135, 185
Medical Device Amendments 68
Medieval era 40–1
menstrual cycle 25, 140–1
menstrual health 153
microchip 184
microscope 17–18
Minos, King of Crete 20, 117
Mirena 128, see also IUD
Mississippi appendectomy 95
Mississippi State Department of Health 9–10
moral acceptability of birth control 35, 39, 57
multipurpose prevention technology 179–81

National Women's Health Network 102, 111
National Women's Law Center 156
Native American 26, 95, 102, 112, 187
Nestorone®/Testosterone (NES/T) 71, 179
Nexplanon, see implant
Nixon, Richard (President) 53–5, 85

noncontraceptive benefits 147–57, 160–2
Nonoxynol-9 (N-9) 179–80
Norplant 105–8, 175, see also implant
Nuremberg Trials 65
Nurses' Health Study 150

obscenity laws 44–9, see also Comstock Acts
Office of Economic Opportunity (OEO) 89
Onan (Biblical) 36, 61, 140
Opill 118–119, 133, 139
Oxford Family Planning Association Contraception Study 150

papaya 22
Paragard 108, 128–9, 178, see also IUD
patch, contraceptive
  as a birth control method 85, 118, 133–4
  breastfeeding and 142
  future 180–3
  prevalence 4
  side effects and benefits 138, 148–60
pelvic inflammatory disease 68, 105, 133
pennyroyal 20, 42
perimenopause 155
period symptoms 150–61
Persephone 15–17
pessary 19, see also diaphragm
pharmacist-prescribed birth control 120
Phexxi (vaginal gel) 137, 178, 180
pill, oral contraceptive
  as a birth control method 132–3
  breastfeeding and 142

future 180–2
history of development 73–87
prevalence 4, 73, 83
side effects and benefits 138, 148–60
Pincus, Gregory Dr. 78–82
Plan B, *see* emergency contraception
Polycystic Ovary Syndrome (PCOS) 126
pomegranate 15–17, 20
Pope John XXI (Peter of Spain) 33, 40
Pope Paul VI 38, 53
Pope Pius XI 37
population control 51–2
Population Council 69, 178–81
poverty
  birth control and poverty reduction 85, 105, 175–6
  eugenics and 91, 95
pregnancy
  ambivalence about 3, 116
  pregnancy-related death (*see* maternal morality)
  unintended 57, 109, 116, 118
premenstrual dysphoric disorder (PMDD) 157, 160
premenstrual syndrome (PMS) 157, 160
Puerto Rico pill trials 65, 80–3

racism 89–113, 187
Reagan, Ronald (President) 53–6
Relf, Mary Alice 89–90, 93–7, 101
religion
  Anglican Church 37
  Buddhism 34
  Catholicism 36–40, 53–54, 81, 120
  Christianity 36–8
  Hinduism 22, 34
  influence of religion on daily life 56–7
  Islam 36
  Judaism 35–6
  Protestantism 37–8
removal of IUDs and implants 121
reproductive coercion 122, 184
reproductive justice 101–13, 115–24, 190, *see also* SisterSong
return to fertility 130–2
right to privacy 10, 48–9, *see also Roe v. Wad*
ring, contraceptive
  breastfeeding and 142
  future 178–83
  historical 27
  as a method of birth control 118, 126–7, 134
  prevalence 4
  side effects and benefits 138, 148–60
Rock, John Dr. 80–3
Roe v. Wade 9–14, 48–9, 122
Royal College of General Practitioners' Oral Contraception Study 149

Saint Augustine 37
Sanger, Margaret 47, 73–80
Second Great Awakening 44
sexually transmitted infections/STI 3, 160–2, 179–81, *see also* HIV; HPV
side effects 157–9
silphium 20–1
Sims, James Marion Dr. 103–5
SisterSong 111, 113, 190, *see also* reproductive Justice
Skyla 129, *see also* IUD
Southern Poverty Law Center 96
spermicide

future 178–83
historical 20, 27, 42, 47, 118
as a method of birth control 135–7, 139
sponge, birth control 35–6, 136, 139
sterilization
access barriers 117, 119
future 183–4
involuntary 90–9, 111–12, 175
tubal ligation 4, 82, 127–8, 138
vasectomy 4, 60–4, 119, 127–8, 138
Susan Thompson Buffett Foundation 186
syphilis 104, 161

telemedicine 121
Thesaurus Pauperum (Treasury of Medicines for the Poor) 33, 40
Title X 52–5, 85–7, 119–20, 187
traditional Chinese medicine 22–3
transgender 3, 98, 156–7, 161, 174
treatise on the heart 19
Tuskegee Syphilis study 104
Tutankhamun (Egyptian Pharoah) 20, 117

United Nations Population Fund 55
unmet need for birth control 119, 174
US Food and Drug Administration (FDA)
and the Affordable Care Act 119

approval of methods 80–4, 102, 105, 108, 142, 180
drug development process 65–9
male birth control 60–2
US Supreme Court cases
Dobbs v. Jackson Women's Health Organization 9–13, 122–3
Eisenstadt v. Baird 47–9
Griswold v. Connecticut 47–9, 167–8
Roe v. Wade 9–14, 48–9, 122
timeline of major cases 49
United States v. One Package 47, 76

venous thromboembolism (VTE) 158–9
Victorian Era 41–3
Voluntary Motherhood Movement 42
vulcanization of rubber 43, 61

witchcraft 40–1
withdrawal method
benefits 139
as a birth control method 140
historical 23–4, 36, 42, 60–1
prevalence 60
workforce participation 171–3
Wrongful Death of a Minor Act 6–13

Y2K 165
Yunxian, Tan 23